DEPARTM

On the State of
THE PUBLIC HEALTH

THE ANNUAL REPORT OF
THE CHIEF MEDICAL OFFICER OF
THE DEPARTMENT OF HEALTH
FOR THE YEAR 1990

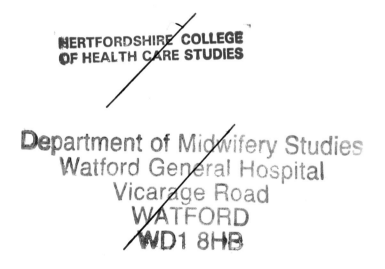

LONDON
HMSO

ISBN 0 11 321435 9

CONTENTS

INTRODUCTION

Rt Hon William Waldegrave MP
Secretary of State for Health

Sir,

I have pleasure in submitting my Report on the State of the Public Health for 1990, together with brief comments on the more important developments and events in the first half of 1991.

The Report is the 133rd in the series since Mr (later Sir) John Simon's first Report for the year 1858, and the eighth and last under my own name. As has been the custom of my predecessors, I give prominence in my introductory chapter both to trends which show progress towards better health and to unsolved problems, or, to use Simon's own words in his first Report to the Privy Council, I "present an account of what has been done, and a comparative gauge of what is required to be done"[1]. On this occasion I draw particular attention to the substantial further improvement in dental health, to some important improvements in the arrangements for postgraduate and continuing medical education, and to the further work that needs to be done in relation to the prevention of illness and promotion of health in older people, family planning, research into the causes of breast cancer, and inequalities of health. As 1990 was the centenary of the death of Edwin Chadwick, whose work lay behind the creation of the post of Chief Medical Officer, I hope I may be permitted, in addition, to examine some of the events of my period in office against a longer perspective.

Public health has been defined as "the science and art of preventing disease, prolonging life and promoting health through the organised efforts of society"[2], and in that sense the successes and failures of public health have been a dominant and recurring theme of the Reports of my predecessors and myself. It was through the influence of Edwin Chadwick that, in 1846, the office of Medical Officer of Health was instituted and the powerful tool of a published Annual Report placed in the hands of the incumbent of the post.

For the ensuing hundred years the local Medical Officers of Health were the key executives for the improvement of health throughout the country. But, by the middle of the present century, the welcome advent of an increasing range of effective, though often expensive, medical and surgical treatments rightly focused attention on therapy, and in particular on the financing and organisation of hospital care. In 1948, a National Health Service, "for prevention and cure of disease and disability by medical treatment . . . and rehabilitation"[3], came into being, and its work and organisation became major features of subsequent Reports. Medical Officers of Health remained with the local authorities outside this new service until their posts were abolished in 1974.

However, the therapeutic revolution soon proved insufficient in itself to fulfil the expectations of men and women about their health and the avoidance of the consequences of illness. The publication this year of the Green Paper *The Health of the Nation*[4] is in many ways the culmination of a series of events associated with a renaissance of many of the ideas which Chadwick and Simon espoused so energetically 150 years ago.

The 'new public health' was born in Canada in 1974. The publication of the Lalonde Report[5] in that year focused attention on the key influence of personal behaviour on health—smoking, alcohol, choice of diet, physical activity and so on. This, in turn, was soon reinforced by important restatements of the key influence of socio-economic factors and the physical environment, including housing[6]. Next came the formulation by WHO of a universal policy which embraced all these elements, including also the provision of appropriate, accessible primary, secondary and tertiary care of high quality. A key additional feature of this strategy was the need to seek the commitment and involvement of the community if efforts to improve health were to succeed. WHO's 'Health for All' policy was drafted in terms which made it suitable for adaptation to the needs of individual countries, and, in 1985, WHO's Regional Committee for Europe published a document which outlined 38 objectives, each with numerical targets which provided challenging, but achievable goals for all the countries within its area.

In England the last few years have witnessed other evidence of the rejuvenation of public health. Chadwick, who in his own lifetime was frustrated by the ineffectiveness of the administrative machinery, would, I hope, have been interested in the Report *Public Health in England*[2], which was published in 1988 and implemented in 1989. The outcome has included several practical measures: a Health Circular that reminds health authorities of their prime duty to improve health, and the need to direct resources towards that end; and the recommendation that Directors of Public Health (DsPH) should be appointed in every District, and should assess the health needs of the population, develop indicators of the outcome of those services, and, like their predecessors the Medical Officers of Health, publish an Annual Report. More recently, these measures have been powerfully reinforced by the designation under the National Health Service and Community Care Act 1990[7] of District Health Authorities (DHAs) as purchasers of health services for a defined population. A further important recent change has been the strengthening of the role of family doctors in relation to prevention and health promotion.

Just as the sanitary revolution, directed by Chadwick and Simon, depended upon accurate information on patterns of mortality supplied by Dr William Farr and the Registrar General's Office, so will the new strategy for health depend upon a new set of indicators which will measure trends in the factors which determine health and ill health, and the hidden precursors of chronic illness and cancer. For this reason the data available to the Central Health Monitoring Unit, which was set up in 1989, will shortly be extended by material derived from an ongoing national health survey.

For the future, the strategy for health outlined in *The Health of the Nation*[4], subscribed to, as it is already, by the whole Government, improved by public consultation, informed by the results of the national health survey, and empowered by commitment from the general population, holds out the prospect of further real improvements in the health of the people of England up to, and beyond, the year 2000. I have little doubt that both Edwin Chadwick and John Simon would have approved.

The Nation's health

Some recent trends

As we enter the final decade of the century, it may be of interest to consider some of the demographic trends to the year 2000 and beyond, and how they will influence health and health services. The first point I wish to make is that the expectation of life at birth will increase further. Thus, the most recent figures from the Government Actuary's Department and the Office of Population Censuses and Surveys (OPCS) project an increase in males from 73.0 years in 1989 to 75.9 years in 2016, and for females from 78.6 years to 80.8 years. Furthermore, the 1989-based population projections for England show a rise of 18% in the population aged 60 years and over during the same period, amounting in absolute terms by the year 2016 to an increase of about 1,785,000 people, of whom no fewer than 440,000 will be over 85 years-of-age (substantially more than five times the capacity of Wembley Stadium).

These projections emphasise the high priority that should be given now to measures directed to improving the quality of health of elderly people, and to the development of services for them. This is the theme of Chapter 3 in this Report; it is also discussed more fully on page 9, and, as the problem of the so-called 'greying of the population' is a feature of many other European countries, it is a key element of the WHO Regional 'Health for All' policy. Target 4 in this policy has the objective of adding health to life as well as years to life. Unfortunately, OPCS data in Chapter 1 indicate that the substantial recent increases in life expectancy for both sexes have not been matched by increases in life expectancy without disability. According to this assessment, between 1976 and 1988 expectation of life with 'chronic disability' rose from 11.8 years to 13.9 years in males, and from 14.4 years to 16.9 years in females. It now seems likely that a substantial proportion of these disabilities are preventable or remediable, and it is certain that preventive action can still produce benefit during the later years of life.

In my last three Reports I have drawn attention to the apparent rise in mortality in the 15-44 years age-group during the latter part of the 1980s, in contrast to a general decline in mortality at other ages. The figures for 1990 show that there has been a further rise in the death rate in males in this age-group. In females aged 15-44 years, the rate has declined for the second year running, but only to a level which still exceeds that in 1985. Although the changing age structure within the 15-44 years age-group accounts for part of these changes, there is no doubt that there has also been at least a cessation, and in some groups a reversal, of the long-standing decline in mortality which requires explanation. At my request OPCS have carried out more detailed analyses to identify the causes of these trends in the latter part of the decade.

Analysis of the trends between 1984 and 1989 within the 15-44 years age-group demonstrates that it is in those under 40 years-of-age that rises or levelling of death rates have occurred. In the 40-44 years age-group, the long-term decline continued to the end of the 1980s—primarily as a result of diminishing rates of coronary heart disease and lung cancer in males, and coronary heart disease and stroke in females. However, amongst men aged 15-39 years, notable increases have occurred in suicides (and open verdicts)—particularly in those aged 15-24

3

years—and in deaths ascribed to AIDS. Amongst women aged 15-39 years, important contributors to the rise in mortality are cancers of the breast and cervix, open verdicts—most of which are likely to be suicides—and chronic liver disease. Mortality trends in the latter category, which have also risen in men aged 30-44 years, are likely to be related to trends in alcohol consumption. OPCS have estimated that if all the causes of death that increased between the periods 1984-86 and 1987-89 are added, they could account for approximately 1,400 extra deaths among men aged 15-39 years. The equivalent figure for females is about 400 extra deaths. A possible explanation, which deserves urgent investigation, is that a proportion of the excess deaths, particularly in the 'suicide' and 'open verdict' categories, is associated with undisclosed HIV-related disease.

In 1990, infant mortality (7.9 deaths per 1,000 live births) and perinatal mortality (8.1 deaths per 1,000 live and stillbirths) were both the lowest ever recorded in England, as were the neonatal and post-neonatal death rates. However, although both infant and perinatal mortality have declined on average by about 30% during the last ten years, about 8,000 deaths continue to occur in England between the twentieth week of pregnancy and the end of the first year of life, and wide differences between Districts and socio-economic groups remain. The strong relationship between low birthweight and death in the first month of life is emphasised in Chapter 1. To take the extreme example, of babies born weighing less than 1,500 grams (less than 1% of all live births), 1 in 4 die in the first month of life. Low birthweight is predominantly the result of premature birth, for which maternal smoking during pregnancy has been identified as the main causal factor. A new Confidential Enquiry into Stillbirths and Deaths in Infancy in the United Kingdom was announced on 2 July. It is hoped that the organisation and mechanisms will be in place by 1992, that data collection on national samples will commence in 1993, and that the identification of avoidable factors will help reduce mortality.

The principal causes of lost years of life before the age of 65 years are cancers, circulatory diseases, accidents and suicide (see Appendix Table A.3). Together these causes account for about two-thirds of all life years lost under 65 years-of-age. The death rate from cancer in the under 65 years age-group declined by 8% during the 1980s, and considerably more in males than females. The sex difference is largely attributable to a substantial fall of 30% in the rate of lung cancer in men under the age of 65 years, due to historical declines in smoking and cigarette tar yields. Although the overall death rate from lung cancer in females aged under 65 years changed little during the same period, trends in smoking prevalence suggest that a fall will take place soon. However, Appendix Table A.3 indicates that in women other forms of cancer, notably breast, uterine and ovarian, are together more important contributors than lung cancer to overall cancer mortality in younger adults. In 1990, breast cancer resulted in a total of 13,000 deaths in women, of which nearly 5,000 occurred in women aged under 65 years. Indeed, in England breast cancer is the second commonest single cause of death of women under 65 years-of-age, causing almost as many deaths as coronary heart disease. I am concerned to find that an examination of the trends during the 1980s reveals no convincing evidence of a fall in mortality rates for breast cancer in young adults. Although the national breast cancer screening programme will offer a significant reduction in mortality from breast cancer in women screened between the ages of 50 years and 64 years, it cannot at present help younger women. In view of England's very high rate of incidence compared with other countries, *I draw attention to the continuing urgent need for research into the enigmas of this common, distressing and fatal disease, and into the causative factors which are clearly continuing to operate so strongly in this country.*

It has been estimated that as much as 85% of cancer may be potentially preventable. Apart from smoking, which accounts for about one third of all cancer deaths, a variety of other factors have been identified as major causes, diet being potentially the most important. In a recent review it was suggested that between 20% and 60% of cancer mortality may be associated with diet, the best estimate being 35%[8]. Many elements of diet have been implicated, although the evidence is sometimes conflicting. There is, however, firm evidence that fruit and green vegetables reduce the risk of stomach cancer; and substantial evidence that 'yellow-green' vegetables reduce the risk of colo-rectal and possibly other cancers. Obesity increases the risk of cancer of the body of the uterus and the gall-bladder, and overweight, whether due to excess total calories or fat, may be related to other cancers, including breast cancer fatality in later life. The potential scope for reducing the toll of cancer deaths related to diet is great. Sufficient evidence about the relationship between dietary factors and cancer is now available to reinforce the advice given on other grounds that the population should increase its consumption of fresh fruit and vegetables, reduce the intake of fat and avoid becoming overweight.

Mortality from coronary heart disease and stroke in those under 65 years-of-age declined throughout the 1980s, falling 27% and 32% respectively between 1980 and 1989. However, deaths in this age-group from these two causes still number over 27,500, and, even if the current rate of decline continues, these two diseases will remain major causes of premature death and illness for many years to come.

Although England's record for accident mortality is one of the best in Europe and is generally improving, there is no room for complacency. In 1990, there were almost 11,000 deaths due to accidents, including more than 600 in those aged under 15 years, of which about half were due to motor vehicle traffic accidents. In childhood, the majority of such fatal traffic accidents involve death of pedestrian children. In May 1990 the Government launched a major child road safety initiative, *Children and Roads: A Safer Way*. It provides a focus for concerted action to reduce child road casualties, including traffic calming, 20 mph zones and the education of all road users. If actual reductions in child pedestrian casualties are to be achieved, it is important that the recommendations within this initiative are put into effect.

Fires also remain an important cause of injury and death. Although only a very small percentage of fires result in casualties—less than 3% of those attended by fire brigades—these still represent a major cause of injury and death. Home Office statistics indicate that 769 deaths were caused by fires attended by local authority fire brigades in England and Wales in 1989, and *I draw attention to the fact that, in contrast to most types of accident, there was no clear downward trend in deaths due to fires during the last decade.* Furthermore, partly but not entirely due to more complete recording of less serious cases, the number of injuries (cases where fire brigades recommended that medical advice should be sought) rose substantially from 7,600 in 1980 to nearly 12,000 in 1989. In 1989, almost 50% of the deaths caused by fire were attributed to being overcome by gas or smoke, compared with a third to burns; a further 10% were attributed to a combination of these causes. Being overcome by gas or smoke was also the largest single cause of injury, accounting for 30% of the total. The highest death rates were among young children and the elderly, particularly the very elderly. Indeed, in 1989 15% of all deaths from fires were in those aged 80 years and over. The rate for injuries was also highest in this age-group, but was also high among young adults. *The wider use of smoke detectors would have a considerable impact on the mortality and injuries from fire and smoke.*

Inequalities in health

In his first Report on the State of the Public Health in England in 1858[1], Sir John Simon pointed to "the inequality with which deaths are distributed in different districts", and drew the firm conclusion that the observed excesses in mortality in some districts were due to local environmental (eg ill-ventilated and crowded dwellings) and social (eg neglect of children) deficiencies which could be remedied. Although health in England has improved beyond all recognition since his day, preventable inequalities in health persist.

In my Report for 1989[9], I reviewed England's progress towards achieving the WHO Regional 'Health for All' target for a reduction in inequalities in health of 25% by the year 2000. I concluded that in England, as in many other countries, this highly desirable target was unlikely to be met, and that major inequalities in mortality between Regions and social groups have continued to exist during the last decade across a wide spectrum of diseases. The persistent difference in self-reported illness between manual and non-manual groups was also discussed. In this year's Report, Chapter 1 includes an analysis of the major types of illness which account for these differences. A gradient in prevalence from the professional group (lowest) to the unskilled manual socio-economic group (highest) was found for each of the three most common groups of chronic illness: musculoskeletal, respiratory and circulatory. The steepest gradient among both men and women was for respiratory conditions, and the differentials in smoking prevalence between the social groups are likely to be a major contributor to this.

The relationship between ill health, premature death and social disadvantage in most industrial societies is complex, and the exact mechanisms remain ill-understood. The fact that inequalities are present and probably increasing, not only within the United Kingdom but within other countries with different political philosophies such as Sweden[10, 11] and Finland[12], bears witness to the fact that there is likely to be no simple prescription available for the solution of this problem. However, analysis has shown that the clearest links with the excess burden of ill health are:

- low income;

- unhealthy behaviour; and

- poor housing and environmental amenities.

There is also strong evidence that close interpersonal relationships and social support from friends and relatives may be protective to health, and that isolation and loneliness have the opposite effect.

Analysis of the major advances in health which have occurred since Sir John Simon's first Report shows that these have been associated more often with improvements in social circumstances than with medical advances. Thus, where people are in a position to exercise greater choice in their housing, environment, employment, leisure activity, and consumption generally, this has tended to be beneficial to their health. By contrast, those not able to exercise greater choice because of low income, lack of education or lack of capacity to take the initiative tend to suffer more ill health.

It is now widely considered that success in the reduction of inequalities of health may require simultaneous action embracing the various areas mentioned above. While to specialists in public health the most attractive points of initial attack are health promotion initiatives to reduce risk factors such as smoking, poor diet and physical inactivity, there is a limit to the extent to which such improvements are likely to occur in the absence of a wider strategy to change the circumstances in which these risks arise by reducing deprivation and improving physical environment. Risk factor reduction, education initiatives and an approach aimed to support and promote self esteem and autonomous action among the most deprived groups in the community are thus linked with, and complementary to, economic action itself.

The emphasis placed in *The Health of the Nation*[4] on intersectoral action underlines the fact that many of the policies required to improve health are outside the scope of the Department of Health (DH), and points to a framework for future action which should be more effective in reducing inequalities.

A strategy for health

In June 1991, a highly significant event took place. The Government published *The Health of the Nation: A Consultative Document for Health in England*[4], which sets out proposals for the development of a national strategy for health. The theme is that the best way to improve health is to select key areas where intervention is capable of producing major improvements, set national targets for each of them, define appropriate indicators, and make arrangements for monitoring progress. The style of the document owes much to the approach of WHO in its pioneering work in formulating the 'Health for All' policy.

The document offers for consultation an initial set of key areas and targets, and indicates the sort of action that will be required to meet these targets, both by the National Health Service (NHS) and others. Sixteen potential areas for action, falling into five groups, have been identified. These are causes of major mortality (coronary heart disease, stroke, cancers and accidents); major categories of ill health (mental illness, diabetes and asthma); key risk factors (smoking, diet, alcohol and physical exercise); other areas with considerable scope for improvement (maternal and child health, rehabilitation and the environment); and areas with great potential for harm (HIV infection and AIDS, other communicable diseases and food safety). An interesting feature is the wide range of suggested targets. These include, for example, not only reductions in mortality from particular diseases, and reductions in health damaging behaviours, but specific clinical targets for more effective management of conditions such as asthma and diabetes, and for rehabilitation services.

Although the role of the NHS is recognised as important, both as a provider of health care, and as an advocate for health, it is clear that the NHS cannot by itself secure, or be expected to secure, all the desired improvements in health. These depend not only on health services, but on the environment (including housing), lifestyle and socio-economic factors. Therefore, the document ranges widely and advocates co-operation for health, not only between the departments of central government in Whitehall, but with local government, the NHS, the statutory bodies, commerce and industry, the professions and the voluntary sector.

As success in improving health must depend on achieving general commitment to the strategy, widespread public discussion is essential. Consultation is therefore under way, not only with the professions, NHS management, patients' representatives and other official and voluntary groups, but also with members of the public themselves. It is hoped to publish a White Paper early in 1992. The reception given to the strategy document in Parliament on 4 June suggests that an evolving health strategy is now likely to be a permanent feature of the English scene.

Health monitoring

During the last year the role of DH's Central Health Monitoring Unit has developed. The Unit has contributed epidemiological data to several initiatives within the Department, and, in collaboration with Departmental colleagues and OPCS, provided the greater part of the epidemiological analysis and the graphic material for *The Health of the Nation*[4]. The Unit is developing a wide range of indicators of the health of the Nation, collating existing information and identifying important gaps. As an essential part of the process to fill these gaps, a new programme of health and nutrition surveys is being developed. These are described more fully below.

A major project in 1990 was a review of the health of elderly people, for which an epidemiological overview of relevant health issues was prepared. This highlighted the major impact on quality of life of illnesses which limit mobility, cardiovascular disorders, and impaired sight and hearing; the influence of social factors (eg the effect of home environment on accidents) on health and health care utilisation; and the projected rise in the number of people over 85 years-of-age during the next ten years. It also pinpointed a number of ways in which the quality of health in the elderly can be improved and will be published in late 1991.

The new health survey

Following the publication of *The Health of the Nation*[4], the work with OPCS on the development of a programme of national health surveys has taken on added significance. In what is hoped to be the initial phase, there will be two elements: firstly, an annual survey of health and nutrition concentrating in the first place on cardiovascular disease and associated risk factors; secondly, a series of detailed dietary and nutrition surveys conducted jointly with the Ministry of Agriculture, Fisheries and Food (MAFF). These will be biennial with each survey covering a different age-group. It is hoped to start the fieldwork for the first dietary and nutrition survey of a nationally representative sample of pre-school children in the summer of 1992. It will be conducted in phases over the following 12 months.

A pilot for the general health survey was successfully conducted by OPCS in March 1991. Fieldwork for the first full survey, covering at least 3,000 adults, is planned for the autumn. It will involve a questionnaire and the measurement of height, weight, waist/hip ratio and blood pressure; a blood sample will be taken and analysed for cholesterol, haemoglobin and ferritin. Subject to Ministerial approval and resources being available, it is hoped that the survey will eventually be enlarged to allow comparisons between Regions and social groups, and extended to cover the priorities agreed for a strategy for health. In this way it will become an essential tool in monitoring progress towards the agreed targets.

The health of people in later life

This year Chapter 3 focuses on the health of people in later life, who have diverse needs for health care. Some older people are active and healthy, others are more frail and need greater support and care; they are not a homogeneous group. Whilst, according to a 1984 survey[13], 39% of people aged 65 years and over take no prescribed medication in the 24 hours prior to interview, and whilst 78% of people aged 75 years and over can manage to walk outdoors independently, diseases of the circulatory and respiratory systems, diseases affecting mobility, and mental health problems diminish the quality of life of many. Depression is a serious problem among older people and in London in 1990 was found to affect approximately 1 in 6. Much of this was unrecognised and untreated.

It is important to recognise that older people can benefit substantially from prevention and health promotion programmes. Thus there is now good evidence that older people can reap immediate benefits from stopping smoking; it is also important that they maintain a balanced diet, avoid obesity, and maintain social contacts. Taking regular physical exercise increases well-being, strength and mobility, and, in women, reduces osteoporosis. The 4th Winter Warmth Campaign *Keep Warm, Keep Well* was launched in 1990; it aimed to help vulnerable and older people to keep warm and well during the cold weather. The new contract for general practitioners (GPs), which was introduced on 1 April 1990, includes a requirement that an assessment must be offered annually to all patients aged 75 years and over, and a similar check every three years to patients aged 16-74 years. For the older age-group the object is to identify and reduce risk factors and to assess home conditions; the Medical Research Council is initiating the development of research into the most effective way of carrying out this surveillance. Cost-effective methods of preventing illness and improving quality of life, rather than simply extending it, need to be actively sought and tested. Until now, much research about prevention has excluded people over the age of 65 years, but in future effective health promotion strategies for older men and women will be essential if the growing number of older people are to have a high quality of life.

Dental health

A new dental contract for the general dental services was introduced on 1 October 1990. The objective is to encourage dentists to be responsible for the long-term care of their patients, including not only treatment but also the use of preventive techniques to protect and maintain oral health. The contract includes written treatment plans, emergency cover and free replacement of some items of treatment found to be inadequate (eg fillings) within 12 months of their being provided. It also includes a capitation system of payment for children up to the age of 18 years and, for adults who are registered with the dentist, provision for a continuing care payment which is not related directly to items of treatment provided.

In February 1991 the results of the 3rd decennial Adult Dental Health Survey of the United Kingdom (UK) were published[14]. The fieldwork had been carried out in 1988 and the preliminary results were published in an OPCS Monitor in 1990[15]. The survey shows steady and substantial improvements in adult dental health compared with the previous national surveys. The proportion of adults with some natural teeth rose from 70% in 1978 to 79% in 1988, and is expected to reach 90% by 2008. By that time more than 90% of the working age population should be substantially dentate, with on average 21 or more natural teeth. Between 1968 and 1988 the pool of sound and untreated teeth in England and Wales increased by 65%, from 294 million to 484 million. At the same time the number of decayed teeth fell by 36%, despite a population growth of 11% due mainly to the increasing number of older people. The most dramatic improvements were in young adults.

Lifestyle and health

Smoking and health

I invariably mention smoking in the Introduction to my Report because it remains the largest single cause of preventable death, causing about 110,000 deaths annually (1 in 6 of all deaths) in the UK, equivalent to the mortality of a jumbo jet crash every day. Smoking is also a factor in about one third of deaths in middle age (40-69 years). This year I underline the ill-effects of smoking in pregnancy and of passive smoking, and mention the efforts to help people to give up.

Smoking in pregnancy

In addition to the general risks to health from cigarette smoking, smoking during pregnancy affects the unborn child. The Independent Scientific Committee on Smoking and Health (ISCSH) reported that associations between smoking during pregnancy and increased fetal and neonatal mortality and reduced birthweight have been demonstrated in many studies since the association with low birthweight was first reported in 1957[16]. It also reported that the increase in perinatal mortality is about 28% and that smoking in pregnancy has been associated with retarded physical and mental development in children. £1 million over two years will be provided for a Health Education Authority (HEA) project to discourage smoking during pregnancy.

Passive smoking

The growing awareness of the risks posed by smoking and the diminishing social acceptability of the habit have resulted in the provision of many more smoke-free areas and increasing interest in the effects of passive smoking. In 1988, the ISCSH[16] estimated that non-smokers exposed to tobacco smoke most of their lives have an appreciable increase in risk of lung cancer as compared with other non-smokers. Such exposure results in the occurrence of several hundred lung cancer deaths each year in this country. The ISCSH also reported that among pre-school children there is an association between exposure to environmental tobacco smoke and episodes of respiratory illness. Recent research shows an association between glue ear (otitis media with effusion) in children and parental smoking, and in one study a third of glue ear cases were attributed to the exposure of children to the tobacco smoke of their parents and other people[17]. More recently, evidence is accumulating that passive smoking may also contribute to the development of coronary heart disease. A review of 12 studies estimated the increase in risk of major coronary events, including death from ischaemic heart disease, to be about 25% in both sexes[18]. These findings should be interpreted with caution because they suggest a surprisingly large effect, and further studies are required. In April of this year, a booklet highlighting the effects on health of passive smoking, prepared by a distinguished group of experts under the chairmanship of Professor Wald, was published by the Imperial Cancer Research Fund and the Cancer Research Campaign[19]. Its publication is both timely and welcome.

Giving up smoking

Giving up smoking is the single most effective step an individual can take to improve the quality and length of life[20]. That being so, it ought to be given at least as much attention as such a key life event as marriage. The health benefits are immediate and substantial, and outweigh any risks from the average weight gain of five pounds that may follow[20]. Former smokers live longer than those who continue to smoke; compared with the risk for continuing smokers, the risk of death begins to decline almost immediately after giving up until, after 15 years, it returns almost to that of those who have never smoked. Giving up smoking greatly reduces the risk of dying from cancer compared with the risk for continuing smokers[20]. For example, a 30-50% reduction after ten years' abstinence has been reported for lung cancer, and a 50% reduction after only a few years for bladder cancer[20]. Cervical cancer risks are also substantially lower after a few years' abstinence[20]. Women who give up smoking before becoming pregnant have babies of the same average weight as those born to women who have never smoked[20]. Even after a lifetime of smoking it is not too late to reap some benefit from stopping.

DH is providing financial support for a 3-year project by QUIT, a voluntary anti-smoking organisation, to promote smoking cessation services in general practice. The aim is to encourage GPs to manage such services as effectively as possible, with a special emphasis on smoking and pregnancy. The intention is to enhance the HEA's work on smoking in pregnancy. DH is also considering what steps, other than funding the HEA's programmes on smoking and the QUIT programme, can be taken to increase the support to those who wish to stop smoking.

Alcohol misuse

Of the 37.5 million drinkers in England and Wales, 1.4 million are heavy drinkers. Heavy drinking is defined as over 50 units per week by men and over 35 units per week by women. Recent population studies indicate a variation of alcohol consumption by social class and by socio-economic group, but no consistent overall pattern. However, there is a positive association between household income and alcohol consumption[21,22]. My Report for 1988[23] referred to the consistent positive relationship between the average per capita alcohol consumption, deaths from chronic liver disease, and the price of alcohol in relation to personal disposable income (or affordability). The key significance of this relationship is gaining increasing recognition within the scientific community and elsewhere.

Injuries resulting from accidents are a major health problem in England and Wales, and accidents are the most common cause of death in the 15-24 years age-group[24]. Alcohol is an associated factor in a large number of accidents and injuries[25], and these may follow the injudicious use of alcohol on single occasions (binge drinking). For young people, it is this pattern of drinking which is more likely to lead to accidents or violence, rather than regular consumption over a prolonged period[26]. It is most encouraging to see that, in their Annual Reports, Regional and District DsPH are outlining the significance of alcohol-related accidents and injuries for local health services[27].

Drug misuse

I feel bound to draw attention to the fact that the number of drug misusers notified to the Home Office Addicts Index has continued to increase, and that the number of cases of AIDS amongst drug misusers is rising more rapidly than in any other exposure category. Information from the first full year of operation of the Regional Drugs Databases will shortly become available; these databases have the potential to collect information on a much wider range of drug misuse than the Home Office Addicts Index, which relies on statutory notification by doctors of contacts with patients addicted to opiates and cocaine. A recent evaluation of syringe and needle exchange schemes has emphasised the need for drug misusers to continue to receive advice and information on all those behaviours which risk the transmission of HIV, not only injecting practices but also sexual behaviour[28]. Although notifications to the Addicts Index of cocaine misuse remained at the same level as in 1989 (10% of first notifications), there is continuing concern that these figures may not fully reflect the increasing availability of cocaine and crack observed in some areas. Abuse of amphetamines by injection continues to be prevalent. A recent comparative study with heroin abuse, which shows that amphetamine abusers are both more sexually active and more inclined to share syringes, emphasises the potential for this type of behaviour to spread HIV infection[29]. Finally, I note that the mortality from volatile substance abuse has also increased throughout the last decade; there were around 130 deaths in 1990[30]. Most of the victims were young men under the age of 20 years, and many were apparently experimenting for the first time. There is a trend towards abuse of the more dangerous butane products rather than glue and solvent-based substances, which were the major problem in the earlier years.

AIDS and HIV infection

By the end of 1990 a cumulative total of 3,817 AIDS cases had been reported in confidence to the Communicable Disease Surveillance Centre (CDSC), of whom 2,100 (55%) had died. Nearly a third of all cases was notified during 1990. The detailed breakdown of HIV and AIDS case reports by risk behaviour category is described in Chapter 5. Although there is evidence of continuing transmission between men who have sex with men, it is important to note that the number of heterosexually active people acquiring HIV infection and developing AIDS (including heterosexuals who acquire HIV infection through injecting drug use) appears to be growing faster than that in any other group, albeit from a low base. This trend is supported by the preliminary results of the anonymous serosurvey programme, which was described in my Report for 1989[31]. The results, which were published in May 1991, show the overall prevalence rate of HIV infection in women attending certain ante-natal clinics in Inner London to be 1 in 500, increasing to as much as 1 in 200 in certain Districts. An earlier study from the Institute of Child Health, using surplus infant blood from Guthrie tests, showed a prevalence rate of 1 in 2,000 in women who had been delivered of a live baby in Inner London in 1988/89. Thus, the rate has increased fourfold in the space of two years. The early results of the anonymous unlinked serosurvey in certain genito-urinary medicine clinics in Inner London showed prevalence rates amongst heterosexuals not classified as intravenous drug users of 1 in 500 in women and 1 in 100 in men. Amongst men who have sex with men and intravenous drug users the prevalence rates were respectively 1 in 5 and 1 in 23. Further efforts are therefore necessary to check the spread of this devastating virus within Britain.

As it has been estimated that no fewer than 1 billion people cross national boundaries every year, either on business or on holiday, sexually transmitted diseases such as HIV infection must also be considered in a global context. World-wide the commonest means of HIV transmission is vaginal intercourse, and the situation is deteriorating. Very high prevalence rates of HIV infection have been reported not only from sub-Saharan Africa, but also from parts of South East Asia, including Thailand and India, and from certain inner city areas within the United States. HIV infection is also prevalent among people who have abused drugs by injection in many parts of Europe, including Italy, Spain and the south of France. It is therefore important to reinforce the advice to travellers on how to avoid infection.

Family planning

The data on abortions in Chapter 1 show that in 1989 there were 163,097 abortions performed under the 1967 Abortion Act on women resident in England. This was the highest number ever reported, and an increase of 40,000 (33%) compared with 1980. A recent survey of women having a live birth suggests that the proportion of live births resulting from an unintended pregnancy may also have been increasing in recent years, from 27% in 1984 to 31% in 1989. It is possible to use these figures to estimate the total proportion of conceptions that were either terminated or regarded as unintended. Between 1984 and 1989 this figure rose from 40% to 45%. Thus, almost half of all conceptions in England were in some sense unwanted or unintended. The figures for girls under the age at which sexual intercourse is legal are also worrying. For those under 16 years-of-age the conception rate was 9.4 per 1,000 women aged 13-15 years, a slight increase on the previous years. In 1988, 53% of conceptions in this age-group resulted in abortions, compared with 54% in 1987. *I draw attention to these figures, which I consider to be unsatisfactory.*

The pilot stage of a national survey of sexual behaviour suggests that a substantial minority of people have had sexual intercourse by the age of 16 years, and the majority by the age of 20 years. It also indicates that it is not uncommon to have more than one sexual partner before entering into a long-lasting relationship. When taken in conjunction with the previous paragraph and the spread of HIV infection described on page 13, these findings highlight the urgent need to improve sex education for young people. They also highlight the importance of easy access to effective consumer friendly family planning, particularly for the young.

The NHS's family planning services are provided by GPs and health authority clinics. Increasingly clients have chosen the former, and two-thirds of family planning is now provided by GPs. This trend has led health authorities to examine, and sometimes to reduce, the scale of provision of clinics. However, it is important to recognise the continuing need to offer clients the option of the more anonymous consultation at a family planning clinic (usually with a female doctor) which is preferred by some people. This is of special significance to the young. It is also relevant for the most mobile section of the population, particularly in cities, for whom family planning clinics can also offer ready advice about preventing the transmission of HIV infection. Health authority clinics may also increase the availability of emergency (post-coital) contraception.

On 30 July 1991 the Minister for Health announced that health authorities had been asked to review their family planning services and to ensure effective co-ordination of the services offered by GPs and at health authority clinics. She added that DH would be issuing family planning guidelines late in the year to assist Regions in their planning.

'Health' food supplements

Popular demand for dietary supplements and 'health' foods has grown significantly in recent years. This has attracted the attention of both MAFF and DH for two reasons: concern that particular dietary supplements sold as foods may represent a hazard to health because of inherent toxicity or poor quality; and the potential to mislead consumers that certain products are necessary and/ or beneficial to health when there is no acceptable evidence. Concerns about the safety of various 'health' food supplements were described in my Report for 1989[32], and problems continued to arise in 1990.

Reports from the USA of severe hepatotoxicity associated with self-medication with high doses of slow-release niacin tablets led to the voluntary withdrawal of these products in the UK. As described in Chapter 7, I was advised to caution women who are (or may become) pregnant against high intakes of vitamin A. The frequency with which DH has to take action against individual products is increasing and, for the first time, specific Regulations have been enacted to prohibit the sale of a dietary supplement, L-tryptophan. Furthermore, the

European Commission is likely to propose a draft Directive on 'diet integrators' (dietary supplements) in the near future.

For these and other reasons, MAFF and DH established a joint Working Group on Dietary Supplements and Health Foods in May 1990 to examine the situation in the UK. It comprises officials from both Departments, including experts from the Medicines Control Agency, with responsibilities for medicine, food safety and nutrition.

The Group's Report is likely to be a comprehensive review of the present controls on dietary supplements sold as foods and medicines. It is also likely to consider the market, the current legislative position, the existing data on the toxicity of dietary supplements, and what is known about their composition (particularly in relation to natural toxicants and contaminants); and set out the available data on the use and intake of dietary supplements in the UK. After consultation the Report's recommendations will be considered by the Government.

Acts of Parliament and official guidelines

Legislation

Three important Bills were enacted by Parliament during the period covered by this Report. The first to be mentioned here, the National Health Service and Community Care Act[7], received Royal Assent on 29 June 1990. Throughout 1990 DH and health authorities prepared to implement the NHS reforms; those concerned with the split between purchasers and providers were especially significant. The former category includes GP fundholders, and the latter NHS Trusts, both of which were established for the first time in April 1991. For the first year of the reforms the intention is that purchasers, funded on the basis of their resident/registered populations, should place contracts which do not lead to unforeseen financial constraint on providers. Funds to allow historical referral patterns to continue were therefore provided. Over the next few years there will be a move towards weighted capitation, a population-based funding mechanism, at local level.

The creation of the purchasing role is one of the major challenges of the NHS reforms and, in the second year, there will be scope for purchasers to seek changes in services to meet the health care needs of local populations. In order to do this, DHAs will have to acquire detailed knowledge of their population's health; obtain information on services known to be effective in addressing health problems; define resources; negotiate contracts for services designed to improve health; and monitor quality and outcome of care. Knowledge about the health needs of a population will be a key feature of public health doctors' contribution to purchasing, as they traditionally have a perspective of health care from a population point of view, and the skills to assess information about the epidemiology of disease and the effectiveness of care. During the early months of 1990, DH took a number of initiatives to support work being undertaken at District level (see Chapters 4 and 6); these led to a major conference on *Purchasing for Health* in May 1991 designed to stimulate managers to the challenges. The challenge of developing a population approach to health should not be underestimated.

The community care reforms will be implemented on a phased timetable leading to full implementation in April 1993. The objective is to allow people to live independently in their homes for as long as they are able and wish. Local authorities will act increasingly as enablers and commissioners of services, and Specific Grants have been made available to improve services for drug and alcohol misusers, and for people with a mental illness. Local authorities will be assessing both individual and population needs for social care in parallel with the assessment of health care needs being carried out by the NHS. As many people will require both health and social care, it is important that doctors and other health care workers are adequately involved in assessments for community care in order to ensure that health care needs are met.

The Human Fertilisation and Embryology Bill was enacted in November 1990[33]. Its provisions bring both the creation and use of human embryos in vitro, and the donation and storage of gametes, under legal control. They also cover the status of the embryo outside the body and of individuals born following the use of donated gametes. An independent Statutory Authority will license embryo research and influence relevant clinical work by licensing and by means of a Code of Practice. The Authority includes lay members as well as scientists and doctors; it assumed its full powers on 1 August 1991 and is expected to begin licensing from September. A draft Code of Practice was published for consultation on 21 March 1991. The final version was approved by the Secretary of State in July and laid before Parliament.

During its passage through Parliament the Bill was extended to include important amendments to the Abortion Act 1967[34]. The principal change is that in future most abortions will have to take place by 24 weeks of gestation. However, there is also provision for abortion to be without time limit for grave permanent injury to the life of the pregnant woman and for substantial risk that, if the child were born, it would suffer from such physical or mental abnormalities as to be seriously handicapped. The changes came into effect on 1 April 1991.

The Food Safety Act 1990[35], which came into effect on 1 January 1991, is the Government's primary response to consumer demands for greater food safety. The Act provides comprehensive enabling powers to deal with European Community (EC) issues and with new developments in food technology. The definition of food has been widened to include dietary supplements and water after it leaves the tap. New enforcement powers under the Act substantially strengthen controls over all aspects of food handling. From 1 April 1992, for the first time, most Crown premises which provide food will be subject to legislative control.

There is a new power for Ministers to make Emergency Control Orders when hazards are found in foods; it provides reserve powers to back up existing voluntary procedures on withdrawing hazardous foods from sale. Powers under the Act also allow Ministers to issue codes of recommended practice for enforcement authorities, so that the law will be applied uniformly across Great Britain. The Act creates statutory backing for the role of 'Food Examiner', who carries out the microbiological examination of food and corresponds to the 'Public Analyst', who has an established role in chemical analysis. The statutory function of the Food Examiner enhances enforcement powers related to risks from the microbiological contamination of food. A new defence of 'due diligence' has been introduced, requiring importers and manufacturers prosecuted for alleged offences under the Act or Regulations to demonstrate adequate quality and safety control procedures.

The Act is intended to provide a balance between effective enforcement and recognition of good practice by the food industry. It has been welcomed by enforcement authorities, industry and consumer interests, and will be the main legislative framework of the Government's food safety policy well into the next century.

Official guidelines

International Commission on Radiological Protection—new guidelines

The International Commission on Radiological Protection (ICRP) provides guidance on the use of radiation sources. Its recommendations were last published in 1977, although interim statements clarifying or extending them have been published in the Annals of ICRP. In view of developments in the last few years, particularly those concerned with estimation of the risks associated with exposure to ionising radiation, ICRP has prepared new recommendations.

In early 1990, a draft was released for comment. In the UK, Government Departments, the National Radiological Protection Board (NRPB) and other interested organisations expressed their views, and DH asked the Committee on Medical Aspects of Radiation in the Environment (COMARE) to provide comments. The text was agreed by the Commission in November 1990 and the final recommendations were published in April 1991.

In ICRP's view, new data and new interpretation of earlier information indicate with reasonable certainty that risks of ionising radiation-induced cancer are about three times higher than they were estimated to be a decade ago. This increase required some quantitative changes in the Commission's recommendations. One example is a reduction of the dose limit for occupational exposure. The previous limit of 50 millisieverts (mSv) per year has been reduced to 20 mSv per year, averaged over five years, with further provision that the dose should not exceed 50 mSv in any single year. The limit for public exposure is now 1 mSv per year or, in special circumstances, 1 mSv per year averaged over five years. In general, these limits do not apply to natural sources of radiation or to the exposure of patients to medical sources of radiation. The Commission has also extended its framework of radiological protection. It now covers situations where there is only a probability of exposure, such as accidents and disposal of solid radioactive wastes, and situations where the source is not under control, such as radon in the home.

NRPB will be advising Government Departments on the applicability of the ICRP recommendations to the UK, where current practices already ensure that both workers and members of the public receive annual doses from artificial sources of radiation well below the new recommended dose limits.

Postgraduate medical education and medical litigation

In view of the Chief Medical Officer's role in the fields of postgraduate and continuing medical education and medical manpower, it has been customary over the years for the Introduction to this Report to include comments on the more important developments in these two fields. This year I comment on some recent developments. I also include a note on medical litigation because of its possible future effects on the quality of the service in obstetrics and gynaecology.

Postgraduate and continuing medical education

In 1990, a major beneficial change took place in the arrangements for postgraduate and continuing medical education. On 6 July, the Secretary of State announced that he had accepted the recommendations of my Expert Advisory Group on the way postgraduate medical education should be funded and organised following implementation of the NHS reforms. The key recommendation is the creation of protected budgets for both postgraduate education and continuing education. The Regional Postgraduate Dean will be the budget holder for the former and the Unit General Manager for the latter. Following the issue of an Executive Letter on 12 September 1990[36], Regions have begun work on identifying current expenditure on the direct costs of postgraduate and continuing education. On 7 January 1991, at a conference attended by managers and educationalists, the Department issued a paper setting out the new arrangements in greater detail[37]. It issued a revised edition of this paper in April 1991, together with an announcement of an initial distribution of the additional £5.8 million announced at the conference in January[38].

Joint Working Party on Women Doctors and their Careers

Almost half the doctors now entering the medical profession from the medical schools are women, and yet, as an employer, the NHS has not so far fully adapted to this situation and to the opportunities it affords. As far as training programmes are concerned, these are unfortunately not always adaptable to women's needs, and they are sometimes the subject of discrimination. In January 1991, Mrs Virginia Bottomley, the Minister for Health, announced publication of the Report of the Joint Working Party on Women Doctors and their Careers[39,40]. The Working Party had taken forward some of the original work carried out by Isobel Allen in 1988, which showed that women doctors were frequently unable to achieve their full potential.

The Report proposes practical measures to help overcome the obstacles to equality of opportunity in the medical profession, which result in the NHS failing to capitalise on a major asset and resource. Mrs Bottomley announced that Government support of £1.5 million would be available for some of the suggested initiatives, the most innovative of which is the WIST (Women in Surgical Training) scheme. This aims to increase the number of women in the surgical specialties by giving them support and encouragement, and will be set up jointly by DH and the Royal College of Surgeons. Other recommendations attracting funding from DH included a new scheme for part-time training at registrar level, and a substantial rise in the fee for the non-training Doctors' Retainer Scheme. The Working Party also made recommendations on other aspects of part-time training, and on equal opportunities in appointments procedures. These recommendations will be considered by DH, health authorities and the Royal Colleges during 1991. In addition, job sharing at consultant level is an obvious way of introducing the flexibility of work which is attractive to some women, and further developments in this area should be encouraged.

Medical litigation

Since the mid-1970s there has been a substantial increase in the number of claims of negligence against doctors and health authorities, and a very substantial increase in the size of court awards and settlements. In response to these increases the Medical Defence Organisations found it necessary to raise their subscriptions for professional indemnity from £336 in 1986 to £1,080 in 1988. Eventually it became necessary for DH to introduce, on 1 January 1990, new arrangements under which health authorities took direct responsibility for handling claims of negligence against their medical and dental staff acting in the course of their NHS employment[41]. Following this major change in procedure the Defence Organisations continue to provide cover for hospital medical and dental staff as far as their work outside the NHS is concerned, and for general medical and dental practitioners. In September, the Department issued further guidance on the handling of claims[42].

In December 1990, the Royal College of Physicians published *Compensation for Adverse Consequences of Medical Intervention*[43]; its recommendations included a 'no-fault compensation' scheme for medical accidents. No-fault compensation was also proposed in two Private Members' Bills, both of which failed to make progress. In the Government's view it is preferable to continue to improve the present system for handling claims of negligence. Changes in the legal system currently under way will ease the passage of such claims through the courts, and, in a debate on the Private Member's Bill proposed by Mrs Rosie Barnes, Member of Parliament for Greenwich, the Secretary of State agreed to examine whether a system of arbitration may be offered within the NHS, as an alternative to adversarial litigation. There will be consultation on any proposals later this year.

Also in December I delivered the William Power Memorial Lecture. My subject, 'Are Obstetrics and Midwifery Doomed?', reflected increasing concern about the trends in litigation, and the threat it might pose to the care of women in pregnancy in view of the increasing number of cases concerning children with cerebral palsy. The lecture provided an opportunity to examine the evidence for the belief that events at the time of birth cause cerebral palsy. The many studies that have been undertaken provide no support for the view that care at the time of birth commonly influences the risk of cerebral palsy. There is some evidence that the burden caused by increasing litigation is one of the factors leading to the early retirement of obstetricians. In the United States it has seriously affected the availability of obstetricians and midwives. I suggest that there is a need to convince the medical, nursing and midwifery professions, the lay public, and the legal profession that the causes of most cases of cerebral palsy lie in the ante-natal period, and that cerebral palsy is therefore no longer commonly a medical accident. Therefore, research on the causes of this common and distressing childhood disability should in future be focused on the ante-natal period rather than on delivery.

The Gulf crisis

It has long been recognised that, during a major war, the NHS might be asked to treat military casualties evacuated to the UK. Together DH, the NHS, the Ministry of Defence (MOD) and the Armed Forces have developed plans for such a possibility. Following the announcement in November 1990 of the United Nations deadline for Iraq to withdraw its forces from Kuwait, suitably adapted plans were finalised to provide care in the UK for any British military casualties that might arise should hostilities occur.

The principal features were immediate resuscitation and treatment of the seriously wounded by military medical services in the Gulf and their evacuation, by air, only when clinically stable; return of other casualties to the UK as soon as possible; provision of appropriate primary and secondary care by the NHS once MOD hospitals in the UK were full; and arrangements by the NHS for casualty reception and dispersal based on its existing contingency plans. Guidance was issued to NHS managers, professional staff and press officers, and all National Poisons Information Service centres were advised of the possible effects of chemical warfare.

After the outbreak of hostilities on 17 January 1991, the NHS plans were implemented by activating a network of 14 Regional Control Centres, with Scottish and Welsh equivalents, linked to MOD's Medical Evacuation Cell (in which DH and the NHS were represented) and a DH Contingency Operations Room. Happily hostilities lasted only a few weeks, chemical weapons were not used and there were few British casualties. Nevertheless, a small number of seriously injured servicemen, none of whom were wounded in battle, were evacuated to the UK; two were referred to NHS hospitals for specialist treatment. These arrangements effectively demonstrated the ability of the detailed plans to facilitate rapid access to medical care.

Acknowledgements

Before I lay down my pen, I wish to record that during the last eight years I have received unfailing support from my medical and administrative colleagues, not only in the Department of Health, but also in many other Government Departments, including the Home Office, the Department of Education and Science and the Department of Social Security, with whom I have had the privilege of working. Without their support, it would not have been possible to perform the duties of Chief Medical Officer, and I express my deep appreciation to them.

Finally I wish to acknowledge the help and support given to me by numerous colleagues in the Department of Health and the Office of Population Censuses and Surveys in the preparation of this Report and those of previous years, in particular the Editor and his staff, and the assistance of Her Majesty's Stationery Office, Norwich, which arranged the printing and publication.

I am, Sir

Your obedient servant

ED Acheson

September 1991

References

1 *The Medical Officer of the Privy Council: Report, 1858.* London: HMSO, 1859.

2 *Public Health in England: the Report of the Committee of Inquiry into Future Development of the Public Health Function.* London: HMSO, 1988. Chairman: Sir Donald Acheson. (Cm. 289).

3 Beveridge WH. *Report on social insurance and allied services.* London: HMSO, 1942. Chairman: Sir William H Beveridge. (Cm. 6404).

4 Department of Health. *The Health of the Nation: a consultative document for health in England.* London: HMSO, 1991. (Cm. 1523).

5 Lalonde M. *A new perspective on the health of Canadians: a working document.* Ottawa: Health and Welfare Canada, 1974.

6 Black D, Morris JN, Smith Cyril, Townsend P, Whitehead M, Davidson N. *Inequalities in Health.* London: Penguin, 1988.

7 *National Health Service and Community Care Act 1990.* London: HMSO, 1990.

8 Doll R, Peto R. *The causes of cancer.* Oxford: Oxford University Press, 1981.

9 Department of Health. *On the State of the Public Health: the annual report of the Chief Medical Officer of the Department of Health for the year 1989.* London: HMSO, 1990; 3, 149.

10 National Board of Health and Welfare. *Public health report.* Stockholm: Socialsstyrelsen, 1988.

11 Dahlgren G, Diderichsen F. *Strategies for equity in health and health services in Sweden—some experiences and suggestions.* Background paper for WHO Meeting on Social Justice and Health: Leeds, 1985.

12 Valkonen T. *Trends in socio-economic mortality differences 1971–85. Department of Sociology, University of Helsinki.* Working Paper no 49: Helsinki, 1990.

13 Cartwright A, Smith C. *Elderly people, their medicines and their doctors.* London: Routledge, 1988.

14 Todd JE, Lader D. *Adult Dental Health 1988.* London: HMSO, 1991.

15 Office of Population Censuses and Surveys. *Adult dental health 1988.* London: HMSO, 1990. (OPCS SS90/1).

16 Independent Committee on Smoking and Health. *Fourth report of the Independent Scientific Committee on Smoking and Health.* London: HMSO, 1988. Chairman: Sir Peter Froggatt.

17 Strachan DP, Jarvis MJ, Feyerabend C. Passive smoking, salivary cotinine concentrations and middle ear effusion in 7-year-old children. *Br Med J* 1989; **298**: 1549-52.

18 Jamrozik K. *Passive smoking and cardiovascular disease.* In: Woodward A, Robert L, editors. Pre-conference workshop on passive smoking: 7th world conference on tobacco and health. Adelaide: South Australian Smoking and Health Project, 1990: 13–35.

19 Imperial Cancer Research Fund and Cancer Research Campaign. *Passive smoking: a health hazard.* London: ICRF, 1991.

20 United States Department of Health and Human Services. *The health benefits of smoking cessation: a report of the Surgeon General, 1990.* Rockville, MD: Office on Smoking and Health, 1990. (DHHS Publication no (CDC) 90-8416).

21 Office of Population Censuses and Surveys. *General Household Survey 1986.* London: HMSO, 1989. (Series GHS; no 16).

22 Office of Population Censuses and Surveys. *General Household Survey 1988.* London: HMSO, 1990. (Series GHS; no 19).

23 Department of Health. *On the State of the Public Health: the annual report of the Chief Medical Officer of the Department of Health for the year 1988.* London: HMSO, 1989;44.

24 Department of Health. *On the State of the Public Health: the annual report of the Chief Medical Officer of the Department of Health for the year 1989.* London: HMSO, 1990;47.

25 Royal College of Physicians. *The medical consequences of alcohol abuse. A great and growing evil.* London: Tavistock, 1987.

26 Shanks J. Alcohol and youth. *World Health Forum* 1990; **11**: 235–41.

27 Alderslade R. *Alcohol misuse: a social problem with medical consequences.* Sheffield: Trent Regional Health Authority, 1990.

28 Lart R, Stimson GV. *Not just a syringe-exchange—a study of the organisation, working practices and philosophy of three syringe-exchanges in England.* London: Centre for Research on Drugs and Health Behaviour, 1991.

29 Klee H. *The potential for the sexual transmission of HIV: heroin and amphetamine injectors compared.* Abstract TUD 106, 7th International Conference on AIDS: Florence, 1991.

30 Wright SP, Pottier ACW, Taylor JC, Norman CL, Anderson HR, Ramsey JD. *Trends in deaths associated with the misuse of volatile substances 1971–1989.* London: Department of Public Health Sciences, St George's Medical School, 1991. (Report no 4).

31 Department of Health. *On the State of the Public Health: the annual report of the Chief Medical Officer of the Department of Health for the year 1989.* London: HMSO, 1990;88.

32 Department of Health. *On the State of the Public Health: the annual report of the Chief Medical Officer of the Department of Health for the year 1989.* London: HMSO, 1990; 10, 145.

33 *Human Fertilisation and Embryology Act 1990.* London: HMSO, 1990.

34 *Abortion Act 1967*. London: HMSO, 1967.

35 *Food Safety Act 1990*. London: HMSO, 1990.

36 Department of Health. *Postgraduate and continuing medical and dental education*. London: Department of Health, 1990. (Executive Letter: EL(90)179).

37 Department of Health. *Working for patients: postgraduate and continuing medical and dental education*. London: Department of Health, 1991.

38 Department of Health. *Postgraduate and continuing medical and dental education*. London: Department of Health, 1991. (Executive Letter: EL(91)51).

39 Department of Health. *Women doctors and their careers: report of the Joint Working Party*. Heywood (Lancashire): Department of Health, 1991.

40 Department of Health. *Women doctors and their careers*. London: Department of Health, 1991. (Press Release 91/23).

41 Department of Health. *Claims of medical negligence against NHS hospital and community doctors and dentists*. Heywood (Lancashire): Department of Health, 1989. (Health Circular: HC(89)34; HC(FP)(89)22).

42 Department of Health. *Handling claims of medical negligence*. London: Department of Health, 1990. (Executive Letter: EL(90)191).

43 Royal College of Physicians. *Compensation for adverse consequences of medical intervention*. London: Royal College of Physicians, 1990.

1. VITAL STATISTICS

(a) Population size

The estimated resident population of England at 30 June 1990 was 47,837,000 persons. The increase of 148,000 (0.3%) compared with 1989 continued the recent trend in annual changes. Most of the increase (106,000) arose from natural change (the excess of births over deaths), and the remainder from net inward migration.

(b) Age and sex structure of the resident population

Appendix Table A.1 shows how the size of the resident population in various age/sex groups has changed over recent years. Between mid-1989 and mid-1990 there was a slight increase in the number of children aged under one year. The number of children aged 1-4 years continued to rise. There was also a slight rise in the population of children of school age (5-15 years), the first such increase since 1976. The adult population of working age (16-64 years for men and 16-59 years for women) continued to rise slowly. An increase in the number aged over 30 years was partially offset by a fall in the number aged 16-29 years as the large cohorts born in the 1960s continued to leave the younger age-group. The population at younger pensionable ages (60/65-74 years) again fell slightly, but there was a continued increase in the numbers aged 75-84 years and, particularly, 85 years and over. Between 1981 and 1990 the populations in these elderly groups rose by 17% and 45% respectively. Women continue to account for about two-thirds of all people over retirement age; three-quarters of the population aged 85 years and over are women.

(c) Fertility statistics—aspects of relevance for health care

Total births

Table 1.1 shows that there were 666,920 live births in England in 1990, 18,000 (3%) more than in 1989, and the highest number since 1972. The number of births has increased each year since 1982 (with the exception of 1989, when births fell by 1%) and the total for 1990 continued this upward trend. The total period fertility rate (TPFR), which measures the average number of children that would be born per woman if the current age specific fertility rates persisted throughout her childbearing life, and is independent of the size and age structure of the female population of childbearing age, was 1.85 in 1990, compared with 1.80 in 1989. The TPFR for England has remained below 2.1, the level leading to long-term 'natural' replacement of the population, since 1972.

The number of births outside marriage continued to rise in 1990, accounting for 28% of all live births, compared with 27% in 1989 and only 12% in 1980. Over 80% of this increase in births outside marriage arose from the increased number of jointly registered births to unmarried couples, the majority of whom stated they were living at the same address, and were presumably cohabiting.

Table 1.1: *Number of live births, crude birth rate, general fertility rate, total period fertility rate and number of live births outside marriage, England, 1980, 1989 and 1990*

Year of birth	Live births	Crude birth rate (births per 1,000 population of all ages)	General fertility rate (births per 1,000 women aged 15-44 years)	Total period fertility rate (TPFR)	Live births outside marriage	
					Solely registered	Jointly registered
1980	618371	13.2	64.0	1.87	31220	42193
1989	649357	13.6	62.5	1.80	50239	124788
1990	666920	13.9	64.3	1.84	51429	137119

Source: OPCS

Average age of mother at first birth within marriage and social class (as defined by husbands' occupation)

Between 1980 and 1990 the mean age of married women at first birth increased from 25.2 to 27.2 years, the highest since records began in 1938. Table 1.2 shows that this trend was evident in all social classes (as defined by husbands' occupation). Married women whose husband's Social Class was I or II continued to have the highest mean ages at first birth, and those whose husbands were in Social Classes IV and V the lowest.

Table 1.2: *Mean age of women at first live birth within marriage, according to social class of husband, England, 1980, 1989 and 1990*

Social class of husband	Mean age of women at first birth within marriage		
	1980	1989	1990
All social classes	25.2	27.0	27.2
I and II	27.6	28.6	28.7
III Non-manual	26.0	27.4	27.4
III Manual	24.4	26.0	26.4
IV and V	23.1	25.1	25.3

Source: OPCS

First births within marriage to women aged 30 years and over

First births to women aged 30 years and over are of medical interest in view of the greater likelihood of obstetric problems associated with first pregnancy at this age. Table 1.3 shows that the number of first births to married women in this age-group was over 6% higher in 1990 than in 1989, and nearly 40% higher than in 1980.

24

Table 1.3: *First births within marriage to women aged 30 years and over, England, 1980, 1989 and 1990*

Age of mother	Number of births (thousands)		
	1980	1989	1990
All ages 30 and over	33.2	43.6	46.4
30-34	27.5	34.2	36.6
35-39	5.0	8.3	8.7
40-44	0.6	1.1	1.2
45 and over	0.1	0.0	0.0

Source: OPCS

Multiple births

Although multiple maternities form only 1% of all maternities, the number has risen steadily over the past decade[1]. Table 1.4 shows that between 1980 and 1990 there was an increase from 6,061 to 7,732. Of the latter, 199 maternities resulted in triplets or higher order births, an increase of 7% compared with 1989 and more than double the number in 1980. Much of this increase is thought to be due to an increased use of fertility drugs and other procedures to assist conception. Figures produced by the Interim Licensing Authority for human fertilisation and embryology show that, in the United Kingdom (UK), there were 62 triplet pregnancies conceived as a result of in vitro fertilisation procedures in 1989, and 19 as a result of gamete intra-fallopian transfer. However, not all of these pregnancies would have resulted in registrable live or stillbirths.

Table 1.4: *Maternities with multiple births, England, 1980, 1989 and 1990*

Year	Maternities with multiple births			Maternities with multiple births per 1,000 maternities
	All	Twins	Triplets or higher	
1980	6061	5968	93	9.8
1989	7378	7192	186	11.4
1990	7732	7533	199	11.7

Source: OPCS

Place of confinement

Table 1.5 shows that, in 1990, the place of confinement for nearly all maternities was a National Health Service (NHS) hospital, with only 1% of confinements occurring at home. This proportion has remained almost unchanged during the past decade.

25

Table 1.5: *Place of confinement, England, 1980, 1989 and 1990*

Year	Maternities (thousands)	Percentage distribution of maternities by place of confinement			
		NHS hospitals	Other hospitals and maternity homes	At home	Elsewhere
1980	616.7	97.5	1.2	1.3	0.1
1989	644.8	97.8	1.1	1.0	0.1
1990	662.0	97.8	1.1	1.1	0.1

Source: OPCS

Total conceptions

Data on conceptions* to women resident in England relate to pregnancies which led to a maternity or to a termination under the Abortion Act 1967[2], but exclude those leading to a spontaneous or illegal abortion. In 1989, an estimated 819,000 conceptions occurred to women resident in England, an increase of 14,000 compared with 1988 (see Table 1.6). Of these, 42% occurred outside marriage compared with only 26% in 1979. The largest number of conceptions and the highest conception rate were amongst women aged 25-29 years. Table 1.7 shows the Regional variation in conception rates. Rates were highest in three of the four Thames Regional Health Authorities (RHAs) (North East Thames 92, South East Thames 86 and North West Thames 85), while the South Western and East Anglian RHAs had the lowest rates (70 and 71 respectively).

Abortions

In 1990 there were 166,460 abortions performed under the 1967 Abortion Act on women who were resident in England. This was an increase of over 3,000 (2%) compared with 1989, and 44,000 (36%) compared with 1980. Of these, 67% occurred in single women whilst 22% occurred in currently married women.

The percentage of all conceptions which led to a legal abortion rose from 16% in 1978 to 20% in 1988. Since 1978 the proportion of conceptions leading to an abortion has risen among women aged 16-31 years, but has fallen among older women (see Figure 1.1). A recent survey of women having a live birth suggests that the proportion of live births resulting from an unintended pregnancy† has been increasing in recent years—from 27% in 1984 to 31% in 1989. It is possible to use these proportions to estimate the total proportion of conceptions that were either terminated or regarded as unintended (excluding terminations carried out because the child would be born with a serious physical or mental handicap). Between 1984 and 1989 this rose from 40% to 45%. Thus almost half of all conceptions to women in England were in some sense unwanted or unintended.

---

* Date of conception is estimated as occurring 38 weeks before date of confinement.

† A pregnancy about which women replied "No" to the question "So would you say you intended to become pregnant that time or not?"

26

Table 1.6: *Total conceptions inside and outside marriage, England, 1979, 1988 and 1989*

Age of woman	All conceptions			Inside marriage			Outside marriage		
	1979	1988	1989	1979	1988	1989	1979	1988	1989
*Under 16**									
Number	8587	8246	7922	41	28	34	8546	8218	7888
Rate	7.5	9.4	9.5	0.0	0.0	0.0	7.5	9.4	9.4
*Under 20***									
Number	113574	113345	110409	30252	12528	11712	83322	100817	98697
Rate	61.6	66.4	67.4	303.1	267.7	275.6	47.8	60.7	61.8
*All ages****									
Number	730203	804565	818923	537975	471860	472610	192228	332705	346313
Rate	76.7	77.3	78.8	90.3	83.8	84.8	54.0	69.7	71.9

Notes:
*   Rates per 1,000 female population aged 13-15 years.
**   Rates per 1,000 female population aged 15-19 years.
***   Rates per 1,000 female population aged 15-44 years.

Source: OPCS

Figure 1.1: *Percentage of conceptions leading to legal abortion by age of woman at time of conception, England, 1978 and 1988*

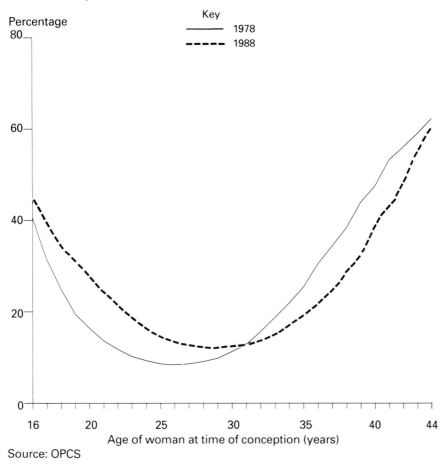

Source: OPCS

In 1990 over 50% of all abortions carried out for women resident in England were on women in their 20s, whilst only 11% were on women aged 35 years and over. The abortion rate was highest among women aged 20-24 years (28.6 abortions per 1,000 women aged 20-24 years).

Table 1.7 shows abortions per 1,000 women for each of the 14 RHAs in England in 1990. The lowest rate occurred in the Northern RHA (10 per 1,000 women aged 14-49 years). In contrast, the highest rates were seen in the four Thames RHAs, where the rate ranged between 16 and 22 abortions per 1,000 women aged 14-49 years. With the exception of the South West Thames RHA, these rates were very much higher than those in all the other RHAs. They may be inflated by women who travel to the South East to have an abortion, and who give their temporary visiting residence as their usual address. The additional cases of abortion may, in turn, inflate the conception rates in the Thames RHAs, which are discussed on page 26.

Table 1.7: *Conceptions, 1989, and live births and abortions, 1990, by Regional Health Authority of usual residence of woman*

RHA of usual residence	Conceptions per 1,000 women* 1989	Live births per 1,000 women* 1990	Abortions per 1,000 women** 1990
Northern	71	62	10
Yorkshire	76	65	11
Trent	73	62	11
East Anglian	71	61	10
NW Thames	85	64	20
NE Thames	92	68	22
SE Thames	86	66	18
SW Thames	79	63	16
Wessex	74	62	11
Oxford	75	62	12
South Western	70	60	10
West Midlands	82	67	14
Mersey	77	65	12
North Western	81	68	12
ENGLAND	79	64	14

* aged 15-44 years.
** aged 14-49 years.

Source: OPCS

Conceptions and abortions to teenagers

The overall teenage conception rate rose from 61.6 per 1,000 women aged 15-19 years in 1979 to 67.4 in 1989. For those aged under 16 years the conception rate was 9.5 per 1,000 women aged 13-15 years in 1989, a slight increase on the previous year. Between 1979 and 1989 there was a notable decrease in the proportion of teenage conceptions that occurred outside marriage and led to a maternity within marriage (from 25% to 7%).

In 1990 22% of legal abortions were on women aged under 20 years; of these 9% were on women aged under 16 years. Over the past decade abortions among women aged under 20 years have risen from 15.0 per 1,000 women aged 14-19 years in 1980 to 20.1 in 1990.

References

1   Botting BJ, Macfarlane AJ, Price FV, eds. *Three, four and more: a study of triplet and higher order births.* London: HMSO, 1990.
2   *Abortion Act 1967.* London: HMSO, 1967.

(d) Mortality

The number of deaths registered in England fell from 539,804 in 1989 to 528,916 in 1990, a decrease of 2%. This resulted in a decrease in the crude mortality rate from 11.3 per 1,000 population in 1989 to 11.1 in 1990.

Figure 1.2: *Excess deaths associated with the influenza epidemic by date of occurrence, Great Britain, November 1989-March 1990*

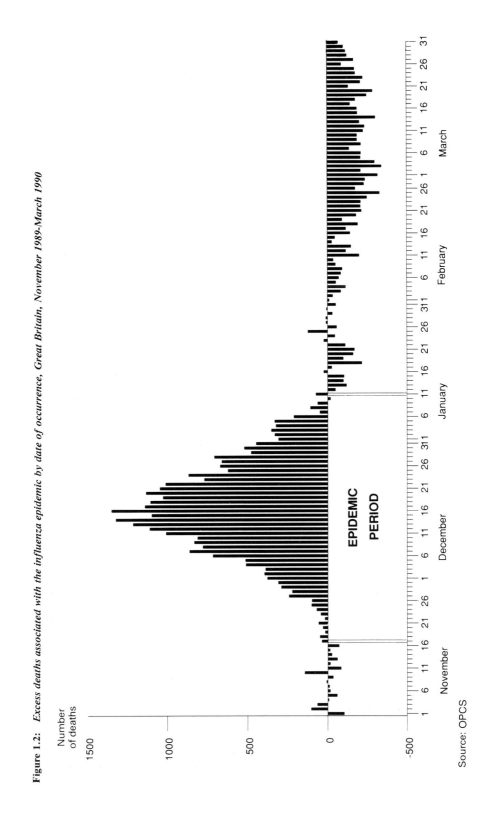

Source: OPCS

Influenza epidemic

The size and course of the 1989/90 influenza epidemic was described in the Report for 1989[1] and reported on fully by the Office of Population Censuses and Surveys (OPCS)[2]. It caused around 25,000 extra deaths between 17 November 1989 and 11 January 1990. More than four-fifths of these excess deaths were of people aged 75 years or more. Subsequent analysis of the epidemic looked firstly at mortality in the weeks following the epidemic. Secondly, it examined all the causes mentioned on death certificates to gain further information about the morbidity of those dying in the epidemic.

From mid-January 1990 daily deaths remained below the expected value for a further three months (see Figure 1.2 and Appendix Figure A.1). The subsequent total deficit over the period up to 31 March 1990 represented only one third of the excess of the previous eight weeks. Only 1 in 10 of the excess deaths was ascribed to influenza on the death certificate. However, more than half of the certificates mentioned a respiratory disease as the underlying or a contributory cause of death. There was also evidence of an increase in mortality among people with mental disease and those with endocrine disorders, principally diabetes. Further details are to be published in *Population Trends 65, OPCS* in the autumn of 1991.

Mortality rates 1980-90

Monitoring mortality during the 1980s has shown that for most age and sex groups death rates declined throughout the decade. However, mortality rates among males aged 15-44 years rose from the middle of the decade, increasing by 4% between 1985 and 1989, and by 5% between 1989 and 1990 (see Figures 1.3 and 1.4). By contrast, mortality among those aged 85 years and over fell by 12% among females and by 17% among males during the last ten years. Mortality rates among children have also fallen in the last decade, although the small numbers of deaths occurring in the 1-14 years age-group have caused fluctuations between years.

Throughout the last decade pedestrian fatalities have been a prominent cause of death among children. Between 1980 and 1990 over half of all deaths from motor vehicle traffic accidents among children were pedestrian fatalities. In 1990 motor vehicle traffic accidents were the second largest cause of death for children aged 1-14 years (see Appendix Table A.2); of these deaths 65% were pedestrian fatalities. However, since 1983 death rates from pedestrian fatalities for children have fallen, from 3.3 per 100,000 population aged 1-14 years to 2.3.

Although motor vehicle traffic accidents are not one of the major causes of death among the elderly, in the last decade they accounted for over 1,000 deaths each year in England among the 65 years and over age-group. Over half of these deaths among males, and over two-thirds among females, were pedestrian fatalities. Between 1980 and 1988 the mortality rate from pedestrian fatalities among the 65 years and over age-group fell, from 15.4 to 10.9 per 100,000 population among males and from 11.8 to 8.4 per 100,000 population among females. In 1990, the rate among females fell further to 8.1, but rose to 11.5 among males. (These data were obtained from death registration statistics and are not comparable with published Department of Transport statistics).

Figure 1.3: *Percentage change in age specific mortality for males, England, 1981-90 (1981 = 100)*

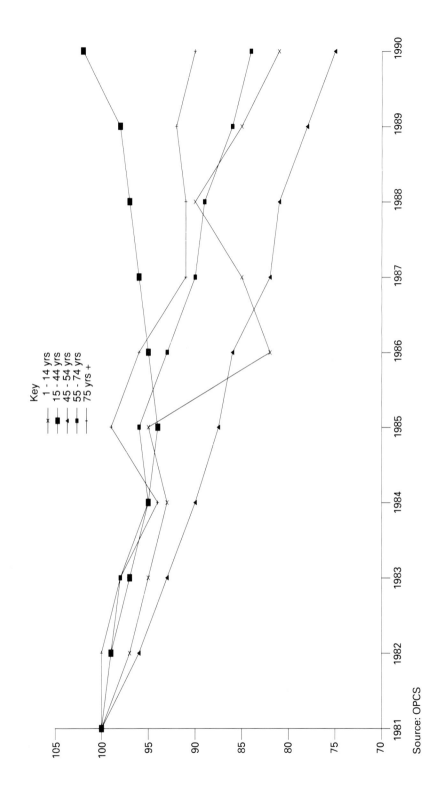

Key
1 - 14 yrs
15 - 44 yrs
45 - 54 yrs
55 - 74 yrs
75 yrs +

Source: OPCS

Figure 1.4: *Percentage change in age specific mortality for females, England, 1981-90 (1981 = 100)*

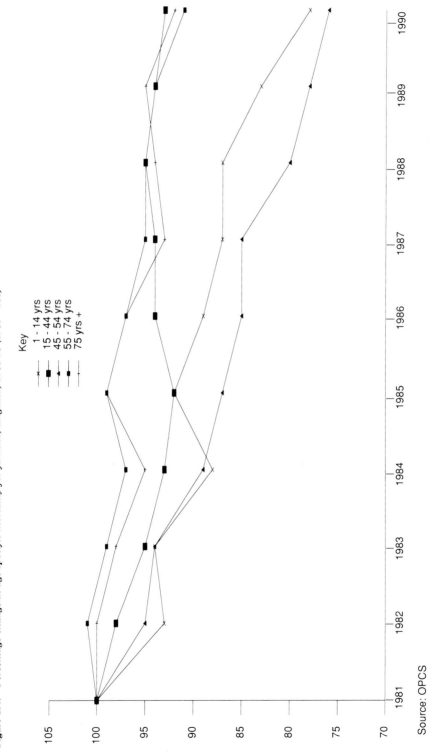

Source: OPCS

Further detailed analysis of deaths among the 15-44 years age-group has continued and will be reported in *Population Trends 64, OPCS* in the summer of 1991. After accounting for the changing age structure within the age-group, death rates for men and women aged 15-44 years levelled between 1985 and 1989 rather than rose as the crude rates suggest. Examination of 5-year age-groups within the age band shows that, for both men and women, the 40-44 years age-group has mortality rates that have continued to decline throughout the 1980s in much the same way as those for the 45-54 years age-group shown in Figures 1.3 and 1.4. When only those aged 15-39 years are considered, each 5-year age-group among women (except the 25-29 years group) experienced a levelling or a rise in mortality rate between the periods 1984-86 and 1987-89. Deaths have been combined for 3-year periods because of the relatively small numbers occurring in these age-groups. Among men, every 5-year age-group has experienced a rise in mortality between the two periods.

Table 1.8: *Increases/decreases in numbers of deaths by cause, 1987-89, compared with expected numbers based on 1984-86 death rates. Men and women aged 15-39 years, England and Wales*

Cause of death (ICD Codes)	Men 15-39	Women 15-39
	Increase/decrease in number of deaths	
Infectious and parasitic (001-139)	24	12
Cancer (140-208)	− 159	
breast (174)		7
cervix (180)		25
other		− 190
Nervous system (320-389)	46	55
Heart disease (410-429)	− 173	− 58
Cerebrovascular disease (430-438)	− 131	− 10
Respiratory disease (460-519)	44	24
Diseases of digestive system (520-579)	4	90
Congenital malformations (740-759)	− 23	3
Accidents (E800-E949)	− 243	− 120
Suicide (E950-E959)	344	− 87
Open verdict (E980-E989)*	476	147
Other including AIDS	438	30
AIDS (279)**	(307)	(24)
Net change in deaths	647	− 72
	(1376-729)	(393-465)

* Injury undetermined whether accidentally or purposely inflicted.
** ICD category 279 is 'Disorders involving the immune mechanism', most of which are AIDS.
Source: OPCS

An analysis of deaths in these 5-year age-groups has been carried out by main causes. The number of deaths occurring in 1987-89 was compared with the number expected based on 1984-86 cause-specific rates. The summary for men and women aged 15-39 years is shown in Table 1.8. In men, decreases in deaths from cancer, circulatory disease and accidents have been more than offset by increased deaths from suicides and AIDS, and deaths of which the cause was an open verdict. If deaths due to all the causes that increased between the two time periods are added together, there may have been 1,400 extra deaths among men aged 15-39 years during the period 1987-89 compared with the period 1984-86. Among women there was a smaller increase of about 400 deaths; these are estimated to have occurred because of increases in deaths from cancer of the breast and cervix, deaths from diseases of the digestive and nervous systems, deaths from AIDS, and deaths of which the cause was an open verdict. The increase noted in deaths from diseases of the digestive system is largely accounted for by increases in chronic liver disease. The death rate for chronic liver disease for women aged 30-44 years increased between 1984-86 and 1987-89, particularly for women aged 35-44 years. For example, the rate for women aged 35-39 years was 14 per million during the period 1978-86. It rose to 30 per million in 1987-89. The corresponding increase for women in their early 40s was from 29 per million to 38 per million. These increases may be related to increased consumption of alcohol by young women[3].

References

1   Department of Health. *On the State of the Public Health: the annual report of the Chief Medical Officer of the Department of Health for the year 1989*. London: HMSO, 1990; 8,17.
2   Curwen M, Dunnell K, Ashley J. Hidden influenza deaths: 1989-90. *Population Trends* 1990; **61**: 31-3.
3   Office of Population Censuses and Surveys. *General Household Survey* 1988. London: HMSO, 1990. (Series GHS no 19).

(e) Infant and perinatal mortality

Infant mortality

Between 1989 and 1990 mortality in the first year of life in England fell from 8.4 to 7.9 infant deaths per 1,000 live births, a decrease of 7%. The greatest decline occurred among post-neonatal deaths, which fell by 8%. The rate fell from 3.7 post-neonatal deaths per 1,000 live births in 1989 to 3.3 in 1990. Infant mortality rates are always higher among males than among females. In 1990 mortality in the first year of life was 8.8 infant deaths per 1,000 male live births and 6.8 per 1,000 female live births.

In the 10-year period 1981-90, infant deaths in England fell by 19% whilst the infant mortality rate fell by 28%. The rate decreased proportionately more than the number because of an increase in the number of live births during this period. Death rates in the first four weeks of life have declined each year during the last decade. The fluctuations in deaths in the first year of life have been determined largely by fluctuations in the death rate for the later part of infancy (post-neonatal)—see Figure 1.5. In 1990, both components of infant mortality—neonatal and post-neonatal—were the lowest ever recorded for England.

Throughout the 1980s sudden infant death was the main cause of post-neonatal deaths in England. It accounted for an increasing proportion of such deaths, rising from 39% of post-neonatal deaths in 1982 to 46% in 1989. Other main causes of post-neonatal deaths in this period were respiratory diseases and congenital anomalies. However, the number of deaths from respiratory diseases more than halved between 1982 and 1989, whilst deaths from congenital anomalies fell by just over a quarter.

35

Figure 1.5: *Deaths in the first year of life, England, 1981-90*

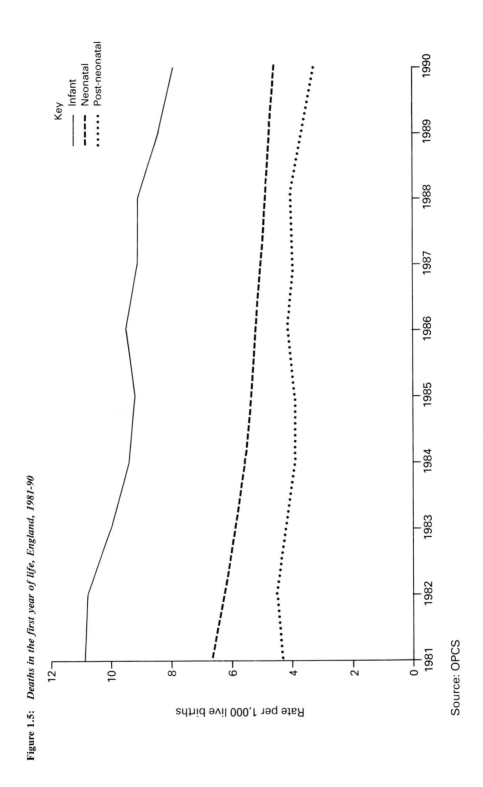

Source: OPCS

Figure 1.6: *Neonatal and post-neonatal mortality rates, and percentage distribution of live births by birthweight, England and Wales, 1989*

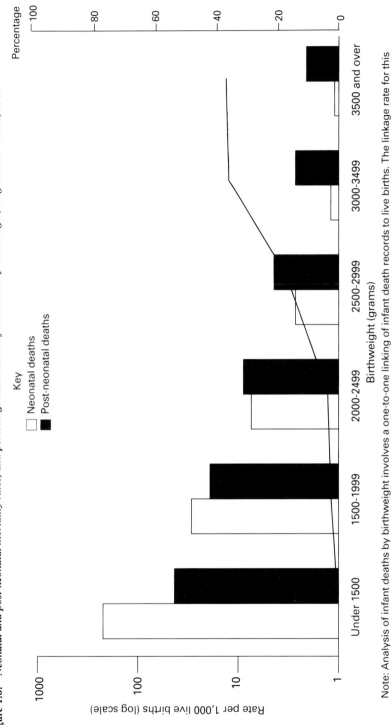

Note: Analysis of infant deaths by birthweight involves a one-to-one linking of infant death records to live births. The linkage rate for this exercise is very high; between 98% and 99% of all infant death records can be linked to the corresponding live birth record.

Source: OPCS

Figure 1.6 gives neonatal and post-neonatal mortality rates for infants of different birthweights, and shows the pronounced relationship between death in the first month of life and birthweight. 1 in 4 babies born weighing less than 1,500 grams dies in the first month of life. A similar but weaker relationship is seen for post-neonatal mortality. The figure also shows the shape and position of the birthweight distribution for all live births. 4 out of 5 babies weighed 3,000 grams or more at birth and these babies had the lowest levels of infant mortality.

Perinatal mortality (stillbirths and deaths in the first week of life)

In 1990, the perinatal mortality rate for England was 8.1 per 1,000 live and stillbirths, a fall of 2% compared with 1989 and 31% compared with 1981. The stillbirth rate fell from 6.5 per 1,000 live and stillbirths in 1981 to 4.6 in 1990.

(f) Acute and chronic sickness

The General Household Survey (GHS) is a continuous survey collecting information about 20,000 adults and 5,000 children in Great Britain each year. It provides two measures of chronic sickness. Firstly, people are asked whether they have any long-standing illness, disability or infirmity. Those who answer "Yes" are then asked "What is the matter with you?", and then whether this "limits their activities in any way". Acute sickness is measured by asking whether in the two weeks prior to interview people had "to cut down on any of the things they usually do because of illness or injury". In 1989, 32% reported a long-standing illness, 18% a limiting long-standing illness and 13% restricted activity in the previous two weeks. Figure 1.7 shows trends from 1979 to 1989 for the three measures for males and females. The rates for acute sickness have changed little, but there is some evidence that rates of long-standing illness have increased during the 1980s. It is not yet clear whether the small fall in prevalence in 1988 and 1989 is a temporary dip.

In 1988 and 1989 answers to the question "What is the matter with you?" were coded. As described in the Report for 1989[1], conditions of the musculoskeletal, circulatory, respiratory and digestive systems were the most commonly reported causes of long-standing illness. The GHS report for 1989 (in press) describes in detail the differences between people in different age, sex, marital status and socio-economic groups. This Report for 1989 drew attention to the continuing differences between manual and non-manual groups in the prevalence of long-standing illness. Data for 1988 and 1989 have now been combined to calculate standardised long-standing illness ratios (SLIRs). These are the ratios of observed to expected prevalence rates, where the expected prevalence rate for a sub-group of the population is obtained by applying the age specific rates for the whole population (of men or women as appropriate) to that group. This ratio therefore removes the effect of the different age structure of sub-groups. Figure 1.8 shows the SLIRs for the three most common chronic diseases for men and women in different socio-economic groups. There is a clear relationship between the prevalence of all three categories of illness and socio-economic group.

Reference

1   Department of Health. On the State of the Public Health: the annual report of the Chief Medical Officer of the Department of Health for the year 1989. London: HMSO, 1990; 25.

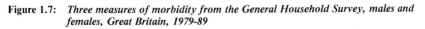

Figure 1.7: *Three measures of morbidity from the General Household Survey, males and females, Great Britain, 1979-89*

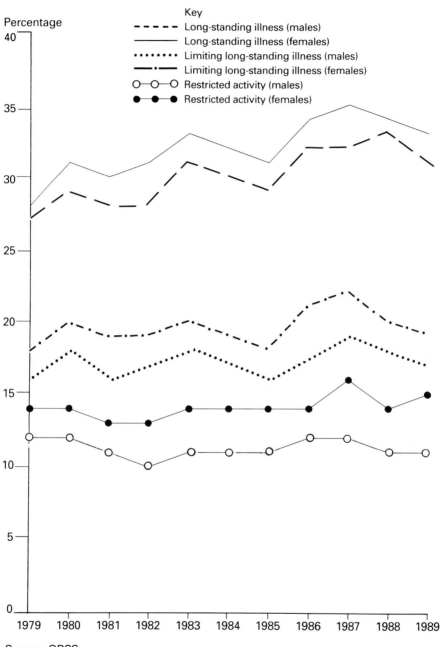

Source: OPCS

Figure 1.8: *Standardised long-standing illness ratios for men and women in different socio-economic groups, Great Britain, 1988/89*

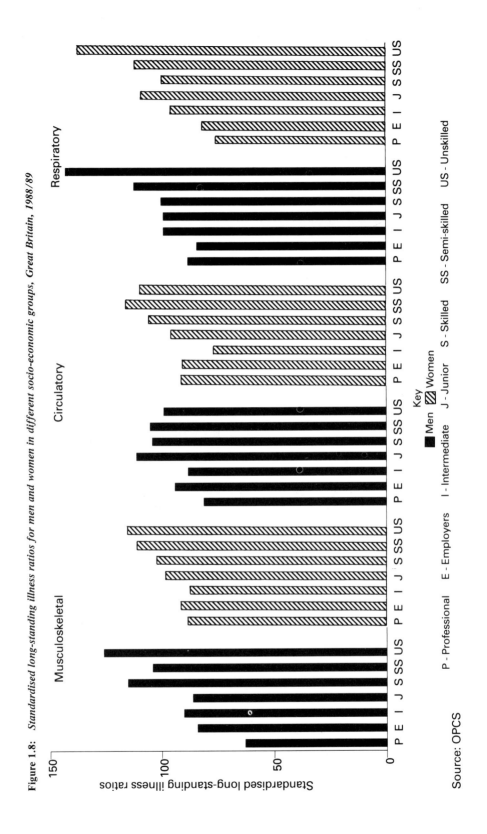

Source: OPCS

(g) Expectation of life without disability

As described in the Report for 1988[1], the prevalence of GHS limiting long-standing illness can be used to calculate expectation of life without disability[2]. This can be used to see if the continued rise in life expectancy, which results from declining mortality rates, has been matched by a corresponding improvement in self-reported health. Figure 1.9 shows trends in both life expectancy and expectation of life without disability. The latter has not improved despite improvements in life expectancy. This suggests that added life years are associated with disability. Similar findings based on the National Health Interview Survey have been reported from the United States[3].

Figure 1.9: *Trends in life expectancy and expectation of life without disability, from birth, England and Wales, 1976-88*

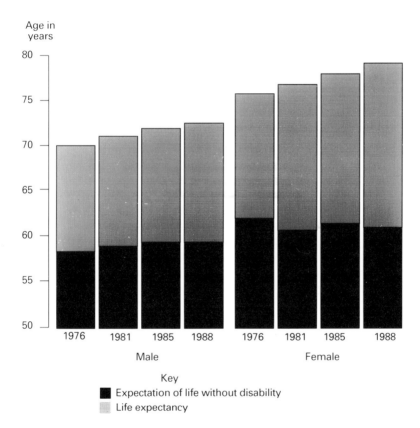

Source: OPCS

References

1 Department of Health. *On the State of the Public Health: the annual report of the Chief Medical Officer of the Department of Health for the year 1988.* London: HMSO, 1989; 27.
2 Bebbington AC. The expectation of life without disability in England and Wales. *Social Science and Medicine* 1988; **27:** 321-6.
3 Crimmins EM, Saito Y, Ingegneri D. Changes in life expectancy and disability-free life expectancy in the United States. *Population and Development Review* 1989; **15:** 235-67.

(h) Trends in cancer* incidence and mortality

Data from the GHS show that 1% of adults reported cancer as a cause of long-standing illness. This estimate can be compared with that based on the OPCS Longitudinal Study, which is discussed in the report of the 1990 review of the cancer registration system[1]. The study brings together, for 1% of the population, information from the national cancer registration scheme, successive censuses and death registration. It suggests that just over half a million people alive in 1981 would have had a cancer registered in the preceding ten years—again a prevalence of around 1%.

The latest national totals of cancer registrations relate to 1986. Appendix Tables A.7 and A.8 show the numbers registered by age, sex and site. They are derived from the latest annual volumes of statistics based on incidence over the period 1977-86. Although the trends must be interpreted with caution, for all cancers together there was no change in incidence during this period. However, when specific sites of malignancy are examined there are some trends of note.

When adjusted for age, lung cancer registration decreased for males but increased for females between 1977 and 1986. For both sexes there was an increase in the number of registrations of malignant melanoma of the skin in 1986 compared with 1985, and there was an overall increase during the period 1977–86. During the same period there was a decrease in registrations of stomach cancer. There were marked downward trends for lymphosarcoma and reticulosarcoma and for Hodgkin's disease, but an upward trend for other malignant neoplasms of lymphoid and histiocytic tissue, to which less well specified lymphomas would be coded. Registrations for cancer of the testis also increased between 1977 and 1986.

The upward trends for bladder cancer and malignant neoplasm of the kidney and other unspecified urinary organs between 1977 and 1984 appear to be levelling off for females. However, the situation is less clear for males. Registrations of carcinoma-in-situ of the cervix uteri were very much higher in 1985 than in previous years, which themselves showed an upward trend, and they were even higher in 1986. However, in respect of carcinoma-in-situ, possible improvements in the level of completeness of registration and in ascertainment need to be taken into account.

As with the incidence of all cancers, there has been no decline in mortality in recent years. Age standardised death rates since the 1920s are shown in Figure 1.10. For men the post-war rise levelled off in the 1970s. For women there was a declining trend until the early 1960s, followed by a rise. Within these totals, however, there was a rise and then a fall in the rate for cancer of the lung/bronchus in men, contrasting with a continuing rise in women. There was a steady fall in the rate for cancer of the stomach in both sexes.

* cancer = malignant neoplasm

Reference

1   Office of Population Censuses and Surveys. *Review of the national cancer registration system: report of the Working Group of the Registrar General's Medical Advisory Committee*. London: HMSO, 1990. (Series MB1 no 17).

Figure 1.10: *Main types of cancer: age standardised death rates per million population by sex, England and Wales, 1921-89*

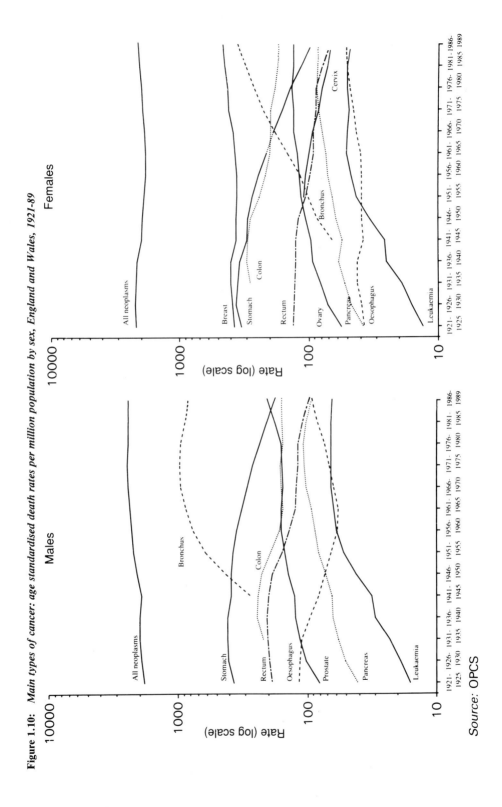

Source: OPCS

43

(i) Appendix Tables and their content (Chapter 10)

Appendix Table 1: Population age and sex structure 1990, and changes by age, England, 1981-90.

This table is described on the first page of this chapter.

Appendix Table 2: Five main causes of death for males and females at different ages, England, 1990.

This table contrasts the major causes of mortality in different age-groups. It should be noted that the rankings are dependent on the particular groupings of disease chosen. Above the age of 35 years, the major burden of mortality derives from circulatory diseases and malignant neoplasms. At ages 15-34 years, road vehicle accidents, other causes of injury and poisoning, and suicide are major contributors to death, particularly in males. These causes of death— other than suicide—are also important in childhood, although congenital anomalies also rank highly.

Appendix Table 3: Relative mortality from various conditions when presented as numbers of deaths and future years of 'working life' lost.

Data presented include the total number of deaths at all ages attributed to selected causes. The percentage distribution of numbers of deaths demonstrates the major impact of circulatory disease and cancer in both sexes. About three-quarters of deaths occur over the age of 65 years.

Data are also presented for years of 'working life' lost between 15 and 64 years in order to indicate the impact of the various causes of death occurring at younger ages. For this tabulation, a death occurring under the age of 15 years accounts for the loss of the full 50-year period between 15 and 64 years, whereas death at age 60 years contributes a loss of only five years of 'working life'. Thus weight is given to the age at death as well as the number of deaths, and emphasis is given to the burden of deaths occurring at younger ages.

In males, although circulatory disease and cancer still contribute substantially to loss of 'working life', other causes become more prominent. These include accidents—mainly motor vehicle—and suicide, and also those of deaths occurring early in life—particularly infant deaths which account for about 20% of years of 'working life' lost. Recent changes in registration procedures preclude presentation of infant deaths occurring under the age of 28 days in this table, although figures for sudden infant deaths—which seldom occur under 28 days—have been included.

In females, the total years of future 'working life' lost from all causes combined is much less than in males, reflecting the considerably lower death rates in females. Cancer—particularly of breast, cervix, uterus and ovary—is a major contributor to loss of life in females aged under 65 years. In 1989, cancer accounted for 24% of all females deaths, but accounted for 38% of years of 'working life' lost. By contrast, although accounting for almost 50% of the total number of deaths, circulatory disease accounted for only 15% of the years of future 'working life' lost. In other respects, the pattern is broadly similar to that for males, although accidents account for a smaller proportion of deaths amongst females.

Appendix Table 4: Trends in 'avoidable' deaths, England and Wales, 1979-89.

The concept of 'avoidable' deaths was discussed in detail in the Report for 1987[1]. These indicators—developed in this country by Professor Walter Holland and his colleagues[2]—have been chosen to identify selected causes of mortality amenable to health service intervention, either preventive or curative. They might best be called potentially 'avoidable' deaths as, while it might not be possible to prevent every death deemed avoidable, it is expected that a substantial proportion could be prevented. The indicators have been made available to health authorities through the Inter-Authority Comparisons and Consultancy (IACC).

The table presents recent secular trends of nine categories of 'avoidable' deaths. The data are presented as age standardised mortality ratios (SMRs), which adjust for differences in the age structure in the years to be compared. During the period 1979-89, declines are evident in all of the categories presented. Cervical cancer and asthma show the smallest declines. Asthma mortality in 1989 was less than in 1979 for the first time since 1980. Trends in asthma morbidity and mortality were discussed in detail in the Report for 1986[3].

Appendix Table 5: Live births, stillbirths, infant mortality and abortions, England, 1960-90.

Secular trends are discussed in this chapter.

Appendix Table 6: Congenital malformations—secular trends in selected malformations, England.

The table presents recent secular trends in the notifications of congenital malformations. The large fall in the numbers of notifications in 1990 is due to the fact that, since January 1990, some minor malformations are no longer reported. The figures for 1990 are therefore not directly comparable with those for earlier years.

Nevertheless this table emphasises the marked decline in malformations of the central nervous system which has occurred in recent years. It is evident in both stillbirths and live births, and probably reflects a decreasing incidence of these malformations. As discussed in the Report for 1985[4], elective abortion following screening is not the major explanation for the decline.

Appendix Table 7: Cancer registrations, England and Wales, 1986 (males).

The table indicates the distribution of cancer registrations in men at different ages. At all ages combined, cancers of the lung, large intestine (including rectum) and skin account for about half of the registrations. In childhood, a high proportion of cancers are attributable to leukaemias, lymphomas, tumours of the central nervous system, and embryonic tumours such as neuroblastomas and retinoblastomas. At older ages, cancer of the lung is the major cause registered. In the oldest age-group presented (85 years and over), prostate cancer accounts for almost as many registrations as lung cancer.

Appendix Table 8: Cancer registrations, England and Wales, 1986 (females).

In childhood, the pattern of female cancers is broadly similar to that in males. However, at ages 25-44 years cancers of the breast (37%) and cervix (18%) predominate. At older ages, breast cancer continues to account for many registrations, although cancers of the lung, skin and large intestine also occur in substantial numbers.

Appendix Table 9: Immunisation in children aged 16 years and under, England, 1976-89/90.

This table is discussed in Chapter 5.

Appendix Table 10: Cumulative total of AIDS cases in England, by transmission category, to 31 December 1990.

Recent trends in AIDS cases are discussed in Chapter 5.

Appendix Figure 1: Weekly deaths, England and Wales, 1989 and 1990, and expected deaths 1990.

This figure illustrates the week-by-week registrations of deaths from all causes at ages one year and over for 1989 and 1990. These can be compared with the expected values for 1990 based on the previous ten years. The sharp rise in mortality observed in late 1989 was due to the influenza epidemic, and has been discussed elsewhere in this chapter.

References

1   Department of Health and Social Security. *On the State of the Public Health: the annual report of the Chief Medical Officer of the Department of Health and Social Security for the year 1987*. London: HMSO, 1988.

2   Charlton JRH, Hartley RM, Silver R, Holland WW. Geographical variation in mortality from conditions amenable to medical intervention in England and Wales. *Lancet* 1983; i: 691-6.

3   Department of Health and Social Security. *On the State of the Public Health: the annual report of the Chief Medical Officer of the Department of Health and Social Security for the year 1986*. London: HMSO, 1987; 24.

4   Department of Health and Social Security. *On the State of the Public Health: the annual report of the Chief Medical Officer of the Department of Health and Social Security for the year 1985*. London: HMSO, 1986; 22.

2. PREVENTION AND HEALTH PROMOTION

(a) Public health in England

Following the Government's acceptance of the main principles underlying the recommendations of *Public Health in England*[1], the Department of Health (DH) issued, in December 1988, Health Circular HC(88)64, *Health of the population: Responsibilities of health authorities*[2]. For the first time health authorities were given the responsibilities of assessing the health needs of their population, allocating resources according to these identified needs, and evaluating the outcome. The circular required health authorities to appoint a Director of Public Health (DPH) to advise them on the discharge of these responsibilities, and the DPH to provide an Annual Report on the health of the local population. That report would be a public document to be presented formally by the DPH to the authority on an appropriate date each year. It would include a core of common data covering the requirements of the Hospital and Community Health Services, the Family Health Services Authority (FHSA) and local authorities. Health authorities were also required to make suitable arrangements for communicable disease control, including the appointment of a consultant with special responsibility for communicable disease control.

In July 1990 Royal Assent was given to the National Health Service and Community Care Act[3]. This Act places a responsibility on health authorities to purchase health care for their population on the basis of identified needs.

Implementation of Health Circular HC(88)64

In accordance with this circular, Regional and District Health Authorities (RHAs and DHAs) had by the end of 1989 completed their reviews of the availability of public health advice, of manpower plans for the specialty of public health medicine, and of arrangements for the control of communicable disease. The Regional reports were varied and were not presented in a common format, making analysis and comparisons difficult. As a result, and in view of the implications of the National Health Service and Community Care Act[3], DH followed-up the implementation of HC(88)64[2] by initiating, in the summer of 1990, a surveillance programme to examine the public health function within the National Health Service (NHS). The objective was to ensure that the spirit embodied in *Public Health in England*[1] was preserved by examining five main areas:

- Directors and Departments of Public Health Medicine.

- Annual health reports.

- Communicable disease control.

- Alliances with Family Health Services Authorities and other agencies.

- Training in public health medicine.

The surveillance programme aimed to cover both qualitative and quantitative aspects. A series of visits to RHAs to collect quantitative data was started, and

47

by the end of the year 9 of the 14 Regions had been visited. A questionnaire designed to provide more quantitative information will be administered in 1991. Work was also undertaken with individual Regional DsPH to examine specific issues.

Directors and Departments of Public Health Medicine

HC(88)64[2] required health authorities to appoint a DPH to advise them on the discharge of their responsibilities. This process was begun in 1989 following the issue of guidance on the appointment of DsPH in June 1988[4]. During 1990, further appointments were made, and by the end of the year 174 Districts had the advice of a DPH. However, there was still a manpower shortage; not all authorities had been able to secure the advice of a DPH and in several cases the arrangements made were temporary. In order to provide advice where DsPH were not available, a number of local arrangements were made, including the sharing of DsPH by Districts. However, even in places where a Director had been appointed, the unavailability of suitably qualified doctors to fill supporting consultant posts in public health medicine was such that many Directors had to continue to work single-handed. To make the best use of the available manpower, there were Regional initiatives to pool skills and encourage co-operation and collaboration between Districts. In some instances Districts worked together in purchasing consortia.

Annual Reports of Directors of Public Health

Following the publication of Health Circular HC(88)64[2], which required District DsPH to publish an Annual Report on the health of their population, an impressive effort was put into the production of these reports across the country. Out of 190 Districts, 111 produced 1989/90 reports by the end of 1990. About 10% of Districts did not have a DPH and so were not obliged to produce an Annual Report.

DH gave advice on the purpose and content of Annual Reports in an Executive Letter[5] and, in the light of the NHS review proposals, consolidated it in a letter from the Chief Medical Officer to DsPH in December 1990[6]. The letter stated that the purpose of annual health reports is:

i.   to inform each DHA, FHSA and RHA about the health of the population for which they are responsible, to report progress, and to identify areas for further improvement, making practical recommendations as far as possible;

ii.   to be an integral component of the health planning and contracting cycle, informing priorities and service specifications; and

iii. to provide information for local authorities, other bodies and the resident population on local health issues.

The letter also stated that "it is important to emphasise that, although the report should be integral to the health planning and contracting cycle, it remains an *independent* report of the District Director of Public Health".

DH commissioned a content review (completed in May 1990) of the first tranche of annual health reports published in 1989/90. The review noted the heterogeneity of the reports and many interesting local highlights. All the reports provided good descriptions of local demography, many referred to WHO's 'Health for All' targets, and a number were enriched with local health surveys.

A number of initiatives to assist the development of annual health reports are under way. Firstly, DH has produced two editions of the *Public Health Common Data Set*[7,8], combining in one place, for each District, a variety of demographic, fertility and mortality information. The third edition will extend the range of information to include some available morbidity information (on cancer registrations, infectious diseases, and congenital malformations), and will also present the information by FHSA area. Secondly, the Faculty of Public Health Medicine has put together a collection of useful information for the compilation of annual health reports. Thirdly, the Royal College of Psychiatrists and the Faculty of Public Health Medicine have organised a joint conference to discuss how to develop the mental health component of future annual health reports (see Chapter 4).

Communicable disease control

The main reason for the establishment of the Public Health Inquiry was the identification of problems concerned with the control of communicable disease. Therefore, as part of the surveillance programme described above (but separate from the main programme), the 14 RHAs were visited between September and December 1990 to ascertain who would be discharging the duties of the Consultant in Communicable Disease Control (CCDC) in each District and his or her professional background, and to identify specific training needs for the competent discharge of the relevant duties. The information obtained will be analysed early in 1991 and form a database for the ongoing surveillance of this important function.

The Regional visits were also used to identify those trainees (mainly in public health medicine and medical microbiology) who might be interested in becoming CsCDC, as a guide to the planning and organisation of relevant training programmes to be provided by Universities, Institutes of Public Health or other educational establishments. Details of existing and planned training programmes were obtained within each Region. These are to be considered by the steering group on training for communicable disease control, which was set up in 1990 by the Faculty of Public Health Medicine, the Royal College of Pathologists, the Royal College of Physicians and a variety of other agencies interested in contributing to such training.

Training in public health medicine

1990 was the second year in which DH provided additional funding for the recruitment of doctors into the specialty of public health medicine. As in 1989, funding was available to increase recruitment to the specialty and to support those who had been appointed the previous year. During 1989 all available posts were filled, and RHAs indicated that they wished to use the additional funding to recruit a further 43 doctors. They also indicated that some of the funding would be required to provide academic and administrative support for a sound training in the specialty.

The Faculty of Public Health Medicine identified the need for further training for consultants already established in the specialty, because of the changing demands being made on the specialty following implementation of the National Health Service and Community Care Act[3]. To meet the identified training needs of consultants, £100,000, to be used in conjunction with RHAs, was made available to the Faculty.

Schools and Institutes of Public Health

The Report for 1989[9] outlined proposals for new Schools of Public Health from eight centres in England which had been tabled at a workshop in London in December 1989, and which were a direct result of recommendations in *Public Health in England*.

Progress has occurred at all eight centres, but at rather different rates as it has been dependent on existing infrastructures, particularly the need for new buildings and the ability to raise funds. Nevertheless, two schools, the School of Public Health in Leeds and the Northern School of Public Health (involving the Universities of Manchester and Salford and Manchester Polytechnic), were officially launched during 1990.

Other centres began operating in a more modest way and on a limited basis. Several made joint appointments with health authorities, usually DsPH, and research posts were also funded. Each has teaching, research and service commitments, although the emphasis differs depending on sponsorship and the centre's constitution. During 1990, proposals for two further schools emerged. In the Trent Region, a school at the University of Nottingham, partly funded by the RHA, is due to open during 1991, whilst in the Wessex Region plans to create an Institute of Public Health Medicine by merging the public health resources of the RHA with those of the University of Southampton are being considered.

Review of the law on infectious disease control

One of the recommendations of *Public Health in England* was that DH "should revise the Public Health (Control of Disease) Act 1984 with a view to providing a more up-to-date and relevant backing to control of communicable disease and infection". A consultation document seeking views on options for change was issued in October 1989[10]. It envisaged that new legislation, covering all aspects of the control of communicable diseases and completely replacing the 1984 Act, would be introduced. More than 500 organisations and individuals submitted replies, many of them lengthy and substantive. The detailed policy is now being developed, and further consultation is being undertaken.

Public health information systems

The NHS reforms have reinforced the need, made explicit by *Public Health in England*, for health information systems to address public health questions and issues. Historically, the provision of such systems was made difficult by NHS Districts being providers of health care and orientated towards catchment populations.

Following publication of the White Paper *Working for Patients*[11], work on information systems culminated in DH publishing *Framework for Information Systems: The Next Steps*[12]. Part I describes changes to be implemented in the short term, ie by 1993. These include a contract minimum data set, and flows of data based on District of residence. There are several references to systems that have implications for health information, for example the setting up of a project to develop an information system for purchasing (District Information Support System (DISS)), an obligation for NHS Trusts to provide information for registers, eg cancer registers, the possible introduction of the collection of data on ethnicity, and the setting up of a project to explore unique patient identification systems. Part II explores some wider and longer term issues which also have implications for health information, for example patient-based systems and record linkage, population registers, medical coding and classification, integration of primary and secondary care systems, and assessments of outcomes. It goes on to describe development and implementation plans.

The development projects that have implications concerning information about health include:

– An extension of DISS to include textual information on policies, effectiveness of services and sources of expertise as well as numerical data, ie the creation of an intelligence function.

– A study commissioned by the NHS Management Executive Information Management Group to consider the corporate needs and demands of the NHS and community services for a Population Health Index and, if it is viable, to consider the options for providing appropriate information systems.

– Various initiatives on medical coding and classification, including preparation for the introduction of the 10th Revision of the International Classification of Diseases (ICD10), setting up an NHS Centre for Coding and Classification (incorporating the Read Clinical Classification System, which now has Crown copyright), and further development of Casemix Classification Systems (such as Diagnostic Related Groups (DRGs)) for use within resource management sites.

In addition, DH commissioned a longer term project, the Public Health Information Specification (PHIS), as part of the work of the Information Management Centre (IMC) in Birmingham. The IMC has been working for several years to produce a Common Basic Specification and Data Models for NHS data.

Following joint work between the Faculty of Public Health Medicine and DH, the Department commissioned the Epidemiology and Public Health Research Unit at the University of Surrey to produce a Public Health Common Data Set. It comprises a series of health indicators, and is used to assist DsPH in the preparation of their Annual Reports on the health of the population. It is issued to DsPH in July of each year, and the 1991 edition will be extended to include some morbidity indicators (see page 49). The data set is now included in DH's Health Service Indicators.

The development of the purchasing function of health and social services authorities, with requirements to assess local needs, to respond to them through the purchase of appropriate cost-effective services, and to monitor their effect in terms of outcome, will bring fresh demands for public health information systems over the next few years.

References

1 *Public Health in England: the Report of the Committee of Inquiry into Future Development of the Public Health Function*. London: HMSO, 1988. Chairman: Sir Donald Acheson. (Cm.289).

2 Department of Health. *Health services management: health of the population: responsibilities of health authorities*. Heywood (Lancashire): Department of Health, 1988. (Health Circular: HC(88)64; Health Circular (Family Practitioner Services): HC(FP)(88)31; Local Authority Circular: LAC(88)22).

3 *National Health Service and Community Care Act 1990*. London: HMSO, 1990.

4 Department of Health. *Appointments to posts in Public Health: Directors of Public Health—consultants in communicable disease control*. Department of Health, 1989. (Executive Letter: EL(89)P/102).

5 Department of Health. *Annual Reports on the Health of the Population*. Department of Health, 1989. (Executive Letter: EL(89)P/13).

6 Department of Health. *Annual Health Reports of Directors of Public Health*. Department of Health, 1990. (Professional Letter: PL/CMO(90)12).

7 Department of Health and University of Surrey: Epidemiology and Public Health Research Unit. *Public Health Common Data Set 1989*. Guildford: University of Surrey, 1989.

8 Department of Health and University of Surrey: Epidemiology and Public Health Research Unit. *Public Health Common Data Set 1990*. Guildford: University of Surrey, 1989.

9 Department of Health. *On the State of the Public Health: the annual report of the Chief Medical Officer of the Department of Health for the year 1989*. London: HMSO, 1990; 36-7.

10 Department of Health. *Review of law on infectious disease control: consultation document*. Stanmore (Middlesex): Department of Health, 1989.

11 Department of Health. *Working for Patients: the NHS review*. London: HMSO, 1989. (Cm.555).

12 Department of Health. *Working for Patients: Framework for Information Systems: The Next Steps*. London: HMSO, 1990.

(b) Smoking and health

Smoking remains the single most important cause of preventable disease and premature death in England[1]. Although the latest available figures (see Table 2.1) show that smoking prevalence continues to fall, the rate of decline is slow and further action is necessary to deal with the problem[2].

Table 2.1: *Prevalence of cigarette smoking in adults (aged 16 years and over) in Great Britain, 1972-88*

	Men %	Women %	Total %
1972	52	41	46
1974	51	41	45
1976	46	38	42
1978	45	37	40
1980	42	37	39
1982	38	33	35
1984	36	32	34
1986	35	31	33
1988	33	30	32

Source: OPCS

Recent reductions in smoking prevalence have occurred in all socio-economic groups, although there is a clear social class gradient (see Table 2.2). Among non-manual workers there is little difference between the sexes in the extent of smoking, but among manual workers the prevalence of smoking is higher among men than women. When both manual and non-manual workers are considered together, there has been a narrowing of the gap between the proportions of males and females smoking since 1972, although the overall prevalence has remained higher amongst men.

Table 2.2: *Cigarette smoking by socio-economic group, Great Britain, 1972-88*

Men	1972 %	1976 %	1978 %	1980 %	1982 %	1984 %	1986 %	1988 %
Non-manual	43	37	36	33	28	28	26	24
Manual	58	52	51	49	44	43	40	40
Women	1972 %	1976 %	1978 %	1980 %	1982 %	1984 %	1986 %	1988 %
Non-manual	38	35	32	32	29	27	26	25
Manual	45	41	41	41	38	37	36	36

Source: OPCS

Lung cancer death rates are related to smoking levels 20-30 years earlier. The rates for men are declining at all ages, reflecting the reduction in men's smoking levels over the past 20 or more years, with reduced tar yields also contributing[3]. The reduction in women's smoking over the same period has been less marked, and lung cancer mortality rates have therefore continued to rise in women aged over 60 years (see Figure 2.1). In younger age-groups the rates among women are showing signs of levelling off. Figures 2.2 and 2.3 show deaths from lung cancer in men and women by health District. The rates for both men and women are higher in the north and west of the country.

Smoking amongst teenagers

A 5-year *Teenage Smoking Campaign*, now in its second year and run jointly by DH and the Health Education Authority (HEA), is achieving remarkably high rates of awareness among its target audience (those aged 11-15 years, particularly girls). The cinema and TV advertising is designed to appeal more to girls and the majority of the press material is carried in magazines for girls. It is, however, too early to identify any positive behavioural changes resulting from the campaign. A major study by the Office of Population Censuses and Surveys (OPCS) into the reasons why children smoke was published during 1990[4]. The report identifies the main factors associated with starting to smoke and will be of great value in determining future strategy.

Passive smoking

There has been growing interest in passive smoking in the last few years; this is leading to an increasing number of controls on smoking in public places, and particularly in the workplace. Several agencies now offer employers advice on the introduction of smoking policies. Parliament has also shown interest in

Figure 2.1: *Trends in death rates from lung cancer, England, 1969-89*

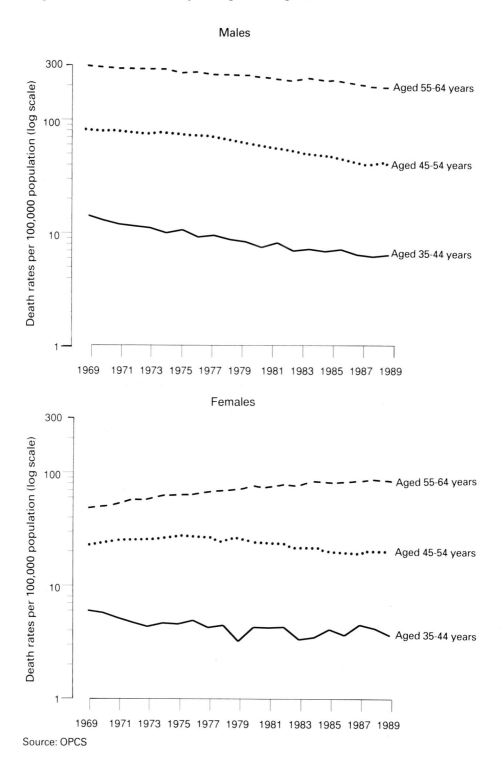

Source: OPCS

Figure 2.2: *Deaths from lung cancer—standardised mortality ratios for males aged over 1 year, England, 1985-89 (England and Wales = 100)*

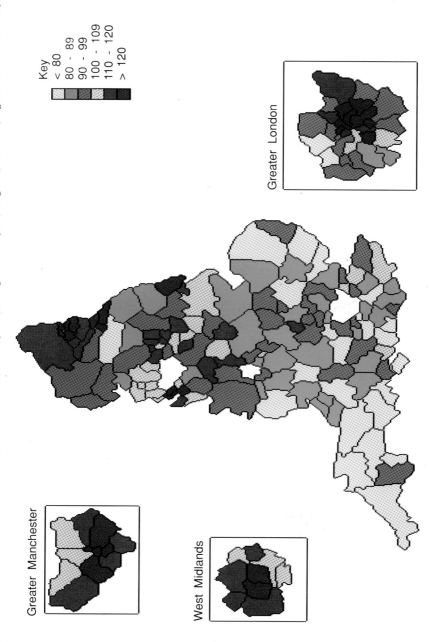

Key
< 80
80 - 89
90 - 99
100 - 109
110 - 120
> 120

Greater London

Greater Manchester

West Midlands

Figure 2.3: *Deaths from lung cancer—standardised mortality ratios for females aged over 1 year, England, 1985-89 (England and Wales = 100)*

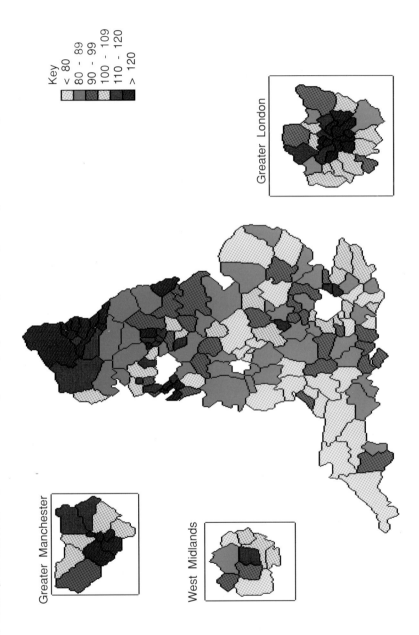

Key
< 80
80 - 89
90 - 99
100 - 109
110 - 120
> 120

Greater London

Greater Manchester

West Midlands

passive smoking, and the *Environment Select Committee Enquiry into Indoor Pollution*, which will be published in 1991, is likely to address this issue. In addition, the White Paper on the Environment contained a commitment on the part of the Government to issue guidance on smoking policies for public places[5]. This guidance is being prepared.

Oral snuff

The Oral Snuff (Safety) Regulations, banning the manufacture and supply of oral snuff in the United Kingdom (UK), came into operation on 13 March 1990. Following an application for judicial review, these Regulations were quashed in December 1990. An appeal against the Court's decision has been lodged.

References

1 Royal College of Physicians of London. *Health or Smoking: follow-up report of the Royal College of Physicians.* London: Pitman Publishing, 1983. Chairman: Sir Douglas Black.

2 Office of Population Censuses and Surveys. *Cigarette smoking 1972-1988.* London: OPCS, 1990. (OPCS Monitor SS 90/2).

3 Independent Scientific Committee on Smoking and Health. *Fourth report of the Independent Committee on Smoking and Health.* London: HMSO, 1988. Chairman: Sir Peter Froggatt.

4 Goddard E. *Why children start smoking: an enquiry carried out by the Social Survey Division of OPCS on behalf of the Department of Health.* London: HMSO, 1990. ISBN 0-11-691327-4.

5 Department of the Environment. *This Common Inheritance: Britain's environmental strategy.* London: HMSO, 1990. (Cm. 1200).

(c) Alcohol misuse

There are about 37.5 million drinkers in England and Wales, of whom about 1.4 million are heavy drinkers[1]. Alcohol consumption in the UK in 1990 was 9.2 litres per head of the population aged 15 years and over. There has been little change in consumption in the last three years.

Social class

A number of recent ad hoc studies and surveys have given some indications of variation of alcohol consumption between social classes. The 1987 OPCS survey *Drinking in England and Wales*[1], which looked at each social class in turn, showed no very clear pattern in average consumption. However, for men there was some evidence of relatively low consumption in Social Class I and high consumption in Social Class V (see Table 2.3). The 1988 General Household Survey (GHS)[2] shows mean consumption by socio-economic group and the pattern is rather different. For both sexes, the percentages of abstainers and very low drinkers rise steadily from the professional group through to unskilled manual workers. For women, the percentage with high consumption falls steadily through the groups. For men, there is no clear pattern of consumption by socio-economic group (see Table 2.4). There is a consistent association between household income and alcohol consumption. As household income increases, members are less likely to be abstainers and more likely to be heavy drinkers. These findings correspond with the general relationship between consumption of alcohol and affordability[3].

Table 2.3: *Average number of units of alcohol consumed in the seven days before interview, by sex and household social class*

All persons aged 16 years and over

Household social class		Units of alcohol	
		Men	Women
I	Professional	11.4	4.3
II	Managerial and junior professional	15.4	6.1
IIIN	Other non-manual	14.0	5.3
IIIM	Skilled manual	15.4	4.6
IV	Semi-skilled manual	12.5	3.4
V	Unskilled manual	17.3	3.7
Total*		14.5	4.8

* The total includes those whose head of household had never worked.

Source: OPCS Drinking in England and Wales in 1987

Binge drinking

Binge drinking is the consumption of a large amount of alcohol on one occasion. Alcohol-related harm may follow not only persistent, regular consumption of alcohol, but also injudicious use of alcohol on single occasions. However, the pattern of alcohol consumption cannot be entirely separated from the level of alcohol consumption, and the more an individual drinks, the more likely it is that some of that drinking will be at the wrong time or the wrong place. Alcohol misuse is one of several factors known to be associated with violent behaviour[4]. Young men aged 18-24 years have the highest proportion of heavy drinkers compared with any other age-group in the population[1]. The average number of units consumed on any one occasion is also greatest in this group[2]. Binge drinking by young men is likely to be at least partly responsible for increasing the risk of being involved in bar fights and sustaining personal injury[5]. Other forms of harm follow binge drinking, and include some road traffic accidents and other accidents.

In 1989, there were 92,820 findings of guilt and cautions for offences of drunkenness in England and Wales. The peak age was 20 years for both male and female offenders[6].

Accidents in which alcohol is a contributory factor

In Great Britain in 1988, there were 22,700 deaths or injuries following road traffic accidents where a driver or rider had a blood alcohol concentration above the legal limit. In addition, 70% of adult pedestrians killed in road accidents at night had high blood alcohol levels. An estimated 840 people died in 1988 in road traffic accidents where at least one driver/rider had a blood alcohol level above the limit[7]. The percentage of drivers killed who were over the legal blood alcohol limit fell from 32% in 1979 to 20% in 1988. The corresponding figures for riders were 31% and 23%. The proportion of drivers and riders involved in accidents resulting in injury and failing a breath test fell from 3.5% in 1979 to 2.4% in 1989[7]. Although care must be taken in interpreting the statistics as the level of police activity influences the number of breath tests carried out, the number of drivers failing a breath test has also

Table 2.4: *Alcohol consumption level by sex and socio-economic group*, Great Britain, 1988*
Persons aged 16 years and over

Alcohol consumption level (units per week)	Professional	Employers and managers	Intermediate and junior non-manual	Skilled manual and own account non-professional	Semi-skilled manual and personal service	Unskilled manual	Total
	%	%	%	%	%	%	%
Men							
Non-drinker	4	5	7	6	9	10	7
Very low (under 1)	5	7	9	11	12	14	10
Low (1-10)	41	37	39	33	33	32	35
Moderate (11-21)	24	23	22	21	20	19	21
Fairly high (22-35)	14 ⎫	15 ⎫	11 ⎫	13 ⎫	12 ⎫	12 ⎫	13 ⎫
High (36-50)	6 ⎬ 25	7 ⎬ 28	6 ⎬ 22	7 ⎬ 29	6 ⎬ 25	6 ⎬ 25	7 ⎬ 26
Very high (51+)	5 ⎭	6 ⎭	5 ⎭	8 ⎭	8 ⎭	7 ⎭	7 ⎭
Base = 100%	576	1786	1413	3042	1240	413	8673
Women							
Non-drinker	8	8	10	11	16	21	12
Very low (under 1)	15	18	21	26	30	34	24
Low (1-7)	43	44	43	39	36	28	40
Moderate (8-14)	19	18	15	14	10	8	14
Fairly high (15-25)	10 ⎫	8 ⎫	7 ⎫	6 ⎫	5 ⎫	5 ⎫	7 ⎫
High (26-35)	3 ⎬ 14	3 ⎬ 13	2 ⎬ 10	2 ⎬ 10	2 ⎬ 8	1 ⎬ 8	2 ⎬ 10
Very high (36+)	2 ⎭	2 ⎭	2 ⎭	2 ⎭	1 ⎭	2 ⎭	2 ⎭
Base = 100%	492	1801	2537	2597	1735	523	10122

* Married women whose husbands were in the household are classified according to their husband's occupation. Members of the Armed Forces, persons in inadequately described occupations and all persons who have never worked are not shown as separate categories but are included in the figures for all persons.

Note: May not add up precisely because of rounding.

Source: OPCS General Household Survey 1988

decreased, although more drivers have been tested. This suggests that fewer people are now drinking and driving, reflecting a success for Government policy in this area.

A significant number of injured people attending Accident and Emergency Departments have positive breath tests[8]; they include many assault victims. Some have established drinking problems, including binge drinking[9]. Alcohol is thought to be a factor in about 15-20% of drownings, and prior alcohol consumption by a proportion of those who die in fires may be a factor affecting their ability to escape[10]. Alcohol has also been linked to domestic accidents[11] and industrial accidents[12].

References

1 Goddard E, Ikin C. *Drinking in England and Wales 1987. An enquiry carried out by the Social Survey Division of OPCS on behalf of the Home Office in association with the Department of Health.* London: HMSO, 1988.

2 Office of Population Censuses and Surveys. *General Household Survey 1988.* London: HMSO, 1990.

3 Department of Health. *On the State of the Public Health: the annual report of the Chief Medical Officer of the Department of Health for the year 1988.* London: HMSO, 1989;44.

4 Substance abuse. In: Blugass R, Bowden P, eds. *Principles and practice of forensic psychiatry.* London: Churchill Livingstone, 1990.

5 Shepherd JP, Robinson L, Levers BGH. Roots of urban violence. *Injury* 1990; **21**:139-41.

6 Home Office. *Offences of Drunkenness, England and Wales 1989.* Croydon: Home Office, 1990. (Statistical Bulletin 40/90).

7 Road Accidents Great Britain 1989. *The Casualty Report.* London: HMSO, 1990.

8 Holt S, Stewart IC, Dixon JMJ, Elton RA, Taylor TV, Little K. Alcohol and the emergency service patient. *Br Med J* 1980; **128**: 638-40.

9 Yates DW, Hadfield JM, Peters K. The Detection of Problem Drinkers in the Accident and Emergency Department. *Br J Addict* 1987; **82**: 163-7.

10 Tether P, Harrison L. Data Note-3. Alcohol-related Fires and Drownings. *Br J Addict* 1986; **81**: 425-31.

11 Royal College of Physicians. *The medical consequences of alcohol abuse. A great and growing evil.* London: Tavistock, 1987.

12 Smith R. Alcohol and work: a promising approach. *Br Med J (Clin Res)* 1981; **283**: 1108-10.

(d) Drug misuse

The total number of addicts notified in England in 1990 was 16,200, a rise of 18% compared with 1989. Of these about 6,300 were first notifications (a 20% increase) and about 9,900 were renotifications (a 17% increase)[1,2]. These large increases may well reflect greater compliance by doctors with the notification requirements and increased success in persuading drug misusers to seek help, superimposed on a continued upward trend in the prevalence of drug misuse. Doctors have recently been reminded of the importance of fulfilling their statutory obligations to notify the Chief Medical Officer of patients whom they know or suspect to be addicted to any of the controlled drugs specified in the Schedule to the Misuse of Drugs (Notification of and Supply to Addicts) Regulations 1973[3,4]. It is vital that doctors should be assured that the highest standards of medical confidentiality apply to the information about drug misusers held on the Addicts Index at the Home Office, and on the new NHS Regional Databases of Drug Misuse. As in previous years, the main drug of misuse was heroin (85% of first notifications); the percentage of addicts misusing cocaine remained the same as in 1989 (10% of first notifications). A major research study on the prevalence of cocaine use among drug misusers, under the supervision of Professor GV Stimson and funded by the Home Office, was started.

The Day report[5] noted that there is major uncertainty about the direction the AIDS epidemic is taking amongst those infected as a result of injecting drug misuse. By 1993, injecting drug misusers, together with those acquiring HIV infection as a result of heterosexual contact, could provide two-thirds or more of new AIDS cases. This possibility emphasises the need for continuing efforts to change the behaviour which puts the drug misuser at risk of HIV infection. Further evaluation of the syringe and needle exchange programmes shows that there are now more than 120 of these schemes, distributing over 4 million syringes and needles each year. Schemes operate from a wide variety of locations, including community pharmacies, drug dependency clinics and voluntary agencies. Research suggests that between 1987 and 1990 drug misusers became less likely to share injecting equipment. Exchange schemes have been successful in attracting drug misusers not in touch with any other services but less so in attracting women, younger drug misusers, certain ethnic minority groups and those at an early stage of drug misuse[6,7,8]. It is now possible to detect HIV antibodies in saliva[9], and a study is under way to obtain, by voluntary testing of saliva, more accurate data on the prevalence of HIV infection among drug misusers attending a range of agencies.

The 1990 phase of the media campaign against drug misuse carried a broad message advising against misuse of a wide variety of drugs, reflecting evidence of the high prevalence of polydrug misuse. There has been growing concern about the extent to which the gel in temazepam capsules is injected by drug misusers. Research suggests an association between high-risk behaviour for HIV infection and the misuse of multiple drugs, particularly temazepam[10]. Temazepam gel-filled capsules have now been reformulated to produce a thicker gel which is more difficult to inject.

General practitioners (GPs) and other doctors outwith the specialist drug misuse services should have an increasing role in providing care for drug misusers, but may lack confidence in their knowledge of how best to meet the needs of these patients. *Guidelines of Good Clinical Practice in the Treatment of Drug Misuse*[11] was distributed to all doctors when it was first published in 1984, and has generally been well received. The guidance would clearly benefit from updating to take account of more recent developments, such as the spread of HIV among drug misusers, and this is now being undertaken.

Under the National Health Service and Community Care Act 1990[12], a new Specific Grant will be payable via local authorities to intitiate, expand or improve voluntary sector provision for drug and alcohol misusers. The Grant, to be introduced in 1991, will support expenditure of £2 million in the first year[13].

Volatile substance abuse

During the 1980s there was an upward trend in deaths from the abuse of volatile substances such as solvents and fuel gases, in spite of measures to educate the public and control supply. Provisional estimates suggest that, in 1990, about 130 deaths in the UK were associated with volatile substance abuse, compared with 82 in 1983 (see Figure 2.4). Most of these deaths were of young people under the age of 20 years; more than 80% of them were male. Glue sniffing and solvent abuse are no longer the main causes of death. Inhalation of fuel gases

Figure 2.4: *Volatile substance abuse deaths, United Kingdom, 1971-90**

Number
of deaths

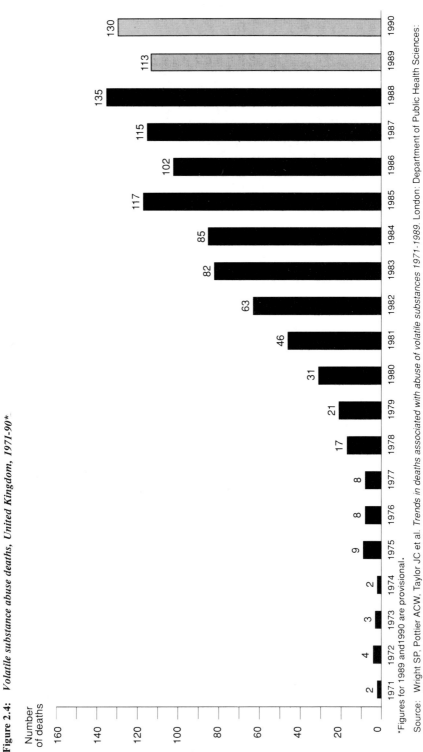

*Figures for 1989 and1990 are provisional.

Source: Wright SP, Pottier ACW, Taylor JC et al. *Trends in deaths associated with abuse of volatile substances 1971-1989.* London: Department of Public Health Sciences: St. George's Medical School. 1991. (Report No. 4)

Figure 2.5: *Volatile substance associated with death by percentage*, United Kingdom, 1971-89*

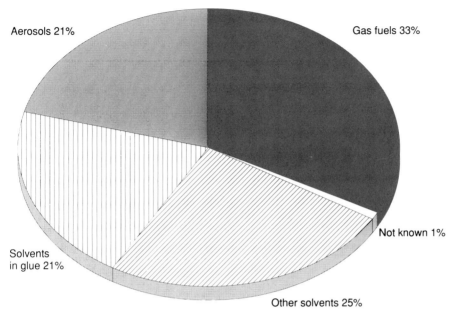

Aerosols 21%

Gas fuels 33%

Not known 1%

Solvents in glue 21%

Other solvents 25%

* Rounded to the nearest integer

Source: Wright SP, Pottier ACW, Taylor JC et al. *Trends in deaths associated with abuse of volatile substances 1971-1989.* London: Department of Public Health Sciences: St. George's Medical School, 1991. (Report No. 4)

such as butane, especially in the form of lighter refills, has emerged as the major problem (see Figure 2.5). Aerosols are the second most commonly abused product. A further demonstration of the dangers of experimentation with volatile substances is that nearly 20% of the deaths due to them between 1971 and 1989 occurred in apparently first-time users. DH provides funding to the National Children's Bureau, to the voluntary organisation Re-Solv, and to maintain a project at the Department of Public Health Sciences at St George's Hospital, London to collect information on deaths associated with volatile substance misuse. The 4th report of the project will be published early in 1991. The statistics now available suggest the need to review what scope exists for further action to reduce this waste of young lives.

References

1 *Data from the Addicts Index January to June 1990.* London: Department of Health, 1991.
2 Statistics of the misuse of drugs: addicts notified to the Home Office, United Kingdom 1990. *Home Office Statistical Bulletin* 1991. London: Home Office, 1991.
3 Acheson D. Notification of drug addicts. *Br Med J* 1990; **300**:1343.
4 *The Misuse of Drugs (notification of and supply to addicts) Regulations 1973.* London: HMSO, 1973. (Statutory Instrument 799).
5 *Acquired Immune Deficiency Syndrome in England and Wales to end 1993: projections using data to end September 1989. Report of a Working Group convened by the Director of the Public Health Laboratory Service (PHLS).* London: PHLS, 1990.
6 Lart R, Stimson GV. National survey of syringe exchange schemes in England. *Br J Addict* 1990; **85**:1433-43.

7   Donoghoe MC, Dolan KA, Stimson GV. *Monitoring Research Group. National Syringe Exchange Monitoring Study. Interim report on characteristics and baseline risk behaviour of clients in England, April to September 1989*. London: Centre for Research on Drugs, 1990.

8   Dolan KA, Donoghoe MC, Jones S, Stimson GV. *A cohort study of clients at four syringe-exchange schemes and comparison groups of drug injectors*. London: Centre for Research on Drugs and Health Behaviour, 1990.

9   Dolan K. Testing saliva for HIV. *Internationl Journal on Drug Policy* 1990; **2** (3):5.

10   Klee H, Faugier J, Hayes C et al. AIDS-related risk behaviour, polydrug use and Temazepam. *Br J Addict* 1990; **85**:1125-32.

11   *Report of the medical working group on drug dependence. Guidelines of good clinical practice in the treatment of drug misuse*. London: Department of Health and Social Security, 1984.

12   *National Health Service and Community Care Act 1990*. London: HMSO, 1990.

13   *Specific grant for making payments to voluntary organisations providing services for alcohol and drug misusers*. London: Department of Health, 1990. (Circulars: HN(90)23, LAC(90)11).

(e) 'Look After Your Heart programme'

The 'Look After Your Heart programme' (LAYH)[1] is England's national coronary heart disease (CHD) prevention programme. It was launched jointly in 1987 by DH and the HEA. LAYH provides information about heart disease and how the risks can be reduced, as well as offering a framework which both encourages and supports action by the individual. In 1990, the LAYH strategy for 1990-95, *Beating Heart Disease in the 1990s*[2], was launched. LAYH continues to develop its role as a national umbrella for CHD prevention activities, providing a common identity to a wide range of national and local initiatives.

Local projects

Local communities continue to play an important part in the work of LAYH. In 1990 the small grants scheme, which supports local heart disease prevention activity, helped fund 56 projects at a cost of £290,000. Also in 1990, a scheme was launched to allow funding of more substantial community-based programmes of up to three years in duration. In 1990/91, £250,000 was provided to fund six large projects, and £140,000 to fund approximately 50 small projects. *Take Heart*[3], which contains examples of good practice in CHD prevention within the community, was published at the end of 1990.

Workplace activities

The popularity of the workplace programme continues to exceed expectations, with demand to join still increasing. Nearly 500 employers have joined the initiative. During 1990, agreement was given to a pilot project to appoint a Regional Workplace Officer in five RHAs.

National promotional activities to raise awareness

During the year LAYH co-operated with the BBC in the production of three television programmes—*Go For It, It Doesn't Have to Hurt,* and *Quit and Win*, which was linked to National No Smoking Day.

September 1990 was *Food for the Heart* month, during which healthy food choices were promoted. Leaflets were jointly produced with Rank Hovis McDougall, and the Meat and Livestock Commission.

Heartbeat Awards Scheme

This scheme is designed to encourage catering establishments to offer a third of their menu as healthy food choices; to ensure a third of their eating area is smoke free; and to have a third of their food handlers trained and qualified in food hygiene. Awards are made with the co-operation of the Institute of Environmental Health Officers (EHOs).

Following a successful pilot scheme, the award was launched nationally with the 1,000th certificate in April 1990. So far 1,643 certificates have been awarded. In the autumn of 1990 a series of seminars for EHOs on the nutrition aspects of the scheme was held and proved to be informative and successful. A directory of establishments which have gained the award will be published in May 1991.

Primary health care

The HEA primary health care unit (PHCU) at Oxford continues to develop the crucial role of primary health care in CHD prevention. In addition to the provision of health education materials, the main areas of work of the PHCU are running multidisciplinary workshops for primary health care teams, providing training for facilitators and health promotion workers, developing a database for general practice, and developing and field testing the 'personal health record'. This is a patient held record card which incorporates health education advice and patient information about lifestyle and risk factors. The PHCU also supports the National Facilitator Scheme, which was set up (with funding from DH) by the Chest, Heart and Stroke Association for the prevention of CHD and stroke.

National Fitness Survey

The Allied Dunbar National Fitness Survey was launched in February 1990[4], with funding from DH, the HEA, the Sports Council and Allied Dunbar (a commercial sponsor). It involves 6,000 adults of all ages answering detailed questionnaires and undergoing a physical fitness assessment at specially designed mobile laboratories. The survey aims to collect 'benchmark' data on who is taking regular exercise, what sort of physical activity is undertaken, and which seems the most effective. The first results are expected in the autumn of 1991.

References

1   Look after your Heart! A campaign to encourage healthier lifestyles in England. *Special Issue Health Trends* 1987; **19** (May special issue).

2   Health Education Authority. *Beating Heart Disease in the 1990s: a strategy for 1990-95*. London: HEA, 1990.

3   Health Education Authority. *Take Heart—good practices in coronary heart disease prevention*. London: HEA, 1990.

4   Allied Dunbar National Fitness Survey. *Project description: a national survey for the Department of Health, the Health Education Authority and the Sports Council*. London: Allied Dunbar, 1990.

(f) Nutrition

The Dietary and Nutritional Survey of British Adults

The first results of this survey, carried out by OPCS in 1986/87 on behalf of both DH and the Ministry of Agriculture, Fisheries and Food (MAFF), were contained in a Report published in June 1990[1]. It contained data never previously available on the diets, heights, weights and blood pressures of a representative sample of British adults aged 16-64 years, as well as biochemical and haematological analyses of blood in those aged over 18 years. This unique wealth of information gave grounds for reassurance on the adequacy of the British diet in relation to most nutrients, but also highlighted a number of areas of concern. 45% of men, and 36% of women, were overweight, with Body Mass Index (BMI)* in excess of 25. Compared with 1980, the prevalence of obesity, defined as BMI in excess of 30, had risen from 6% to 8% of men, and from 8% to 12% of women. 18% of women aged 50-64 years were obese.

The survey involved a weighed record of all food and drink consumed over seven days, and found that average intakes of fat and of saturated fatty acids, at 40% and 16% of food energy, were undesirably high. Only 6% of men and 8% of women met the targets set by the Committee on Medical Aspects of Food Policy (COMA) of no more than 35% of food energy from fat and 15% from saturated fatty acids. Serum cholesterol was found to be above the desirable range (up to 5.2 mmol/litre) in 34% of respondents, a figure which increased with age. Of women aged 50-64 years, 21% had severely elevated levels (7.8 mmol/litre or greater). Although anaemia was very uncommon, 17% of women of childbearing age were found to have low body stores of iron, with serum ferritin below 13 micrograms/litre.

'Eight Guidelines for a Healthy Diet'

DH, MAFF, and the HEA jointly published a booklet entitled *Eight Guidelines for a Healthy Diet*[2]. These guidelines were endorsed by COMA. The booklet explains the basis of healthy eating for the population. Aimed at those in the general population who influence people's eating habits, it provides a robust framework for health professionals and lay people on which to base advice about diet and health, and was accompanied by a brief text which gave simple explanations for the advice, while dispelling some common misconceptions. The impact of this venture is being evaluated prior to considering further, more focused material in the future.

Diet and cardiovascular disease

In 1984 COMA published its influential Report on *Diet and Cardiovascular Disease*[3]. Since then there has been a substantial increase in public interest in the relationships between diet and health, reflected in the media as well as in scientific research. COMA therefore decided to convene a new panel to review the latest evidence on the relationship between diet and cardiovascular disease. Chaired by Professor Michael Marmot, it is expected to report in 1992. Although dietary patterns have altered substantially over recent years, the 1984 targets have still not been achieved[1], and COMA asked the new panel to identify barriers to the implementation of the recommendations in the 1984 Report and to make its own recommendations in this respect. This work is running in parallel with the main review, and is expected to influence the form of the final recommendations.

---

* Body Mass Index (BMI) is calculated by dividing weight in kilograms by the square of the height in metres.

Infant feeding survey 1990

Infant feeding practices have been surveyed nationally every five years since 1975[4]. The fourth such survey was commissioned by DH in 1990. OPCS have asked some 10,000 mothers to complete questionnaires about how their babies were being fed at 6 weeks, and at 4 and 9 months-of-age. The results of the survey are expected in late 1991, and will provide information of value to health professionals and policy makers, in particular on current rates of breast-feeding. For the first time, all UK countries have taken part.

References

1 Gregory J, Foster K, Tyler H, Wiseman M. *The Dietary and Nutritional Survey of British Adults*. London: HMSO, 1990.
2 Department of Health, Ministry of Agriculture, Fisheries and Food, Health Education Authority. *Eight Guidelines for a Healthy Diet*. London: Food Sense, 1990.
3 Department of Health and Social Security. *Diet and Cardiovascular Disease*. London: HMSO, 1984. (Report on health and social subjects no 28).
4 Martin J, White A. *Infant Feeding 1985*. London: HMSO, 1988.

3. HEALTH OF PEOPLE IN LATER LIFE

Introduction

Throughout the last one hundred years, life expectancy has been increasing, and more people than ever before now enjoy a healthy life in their sixties, seventies, eighties and beyond. Once a person has reached the age of 65 years, average life expectancy is now a further 18 years for women and 14 years for men. In the last 80 years, life expectancy in England and Wales at the age of 60 years has increased by over 6 years for women and 3 years for men. There is a wide range in health amongst people in later life, from those who are active and healthy (now sometimes referred to as people in their third age) to those who are frail and need support and care. People in later life have much to enjoy, and much to contribute to society, and they should not be impaired by avoidable illness and disability.

The first section of this chapter presents the recent and continuing demographic and social changes of people in later life. Sections (b)—(e) deal with the health of people in later life and of their carers, section (f) examines the opportunities for the prevention of illness and health promotion, and section (g) rehabilitation. Where possible, the differing circumstances of people aged 65-74 years, 75-84 years and 85 years and over have been considered.

(a) Challenges of a changing population

Within England and Wales in 1990, 13% of the male population and 19% of the female population were aged 65 years or more. Taken as a whole the number of people aged over 65 years is increasing only slowly. However, this slow increase disguises the fact that, whereas there is a decline in the number of people aged 65-74 years, there is an increase in the number in the older age-groups, particularly in those aged over 85 years (see Figures 3.1 and 3.2). The Office of Population Censuses and Surveys (OPCS) estimates that in 1990 there were in England and Wales 776,000 people aged 85 years or more; in the year 2000 this is projected to rise to 1,049,000—an increase of 35%[1]. In the United Kingdom (UK) in 1990, there were approximately five people of working age (15-64 years) for every person aged over 65 years. By the year 2030, this ratio will have declined so that for every person aged 65 years and over there will be only three people of working age.

A second important trend is the projected change in the sex ratio (males per 100 females) in all age-groups, with a higher proportion of men living into later life. Between 1991 and 2001, the projected sex ratio will increase from 79 to 88 for people aged 65-74 years, from 58 to 65 for people aged 75-84 years, and from 34 to 38 for people aged 85 years and over.

Table 3.1 shows the increased proportion of people aged over 65 years who live alone, or with their spouse only, compared with those who live with other family members or friends. A higher proportion of women than men live alone, and this increases with age. Data from the 1986 General Household Survey (GHS)[2] showed that 61% of women aged 85 years and over lived alone compared with 37% of men, and that 33% of women aged 65-69 years lived alone, compared with 13% of men in the same age-group.

Figure 3.1: *Elderly male population: age-group trends, England and Wales,*
1966-2026

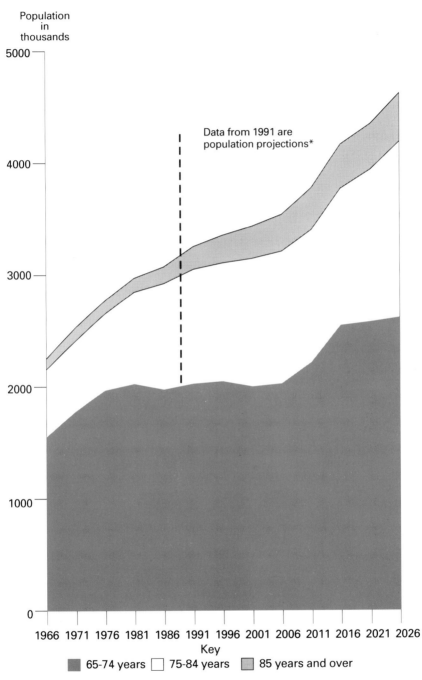

* Based on the Registrar General's mid-1989 estimates.

Source: OPCS

Figure 3.2: *Elderly female population: age-group trends, England and Wales, 1966-2026*

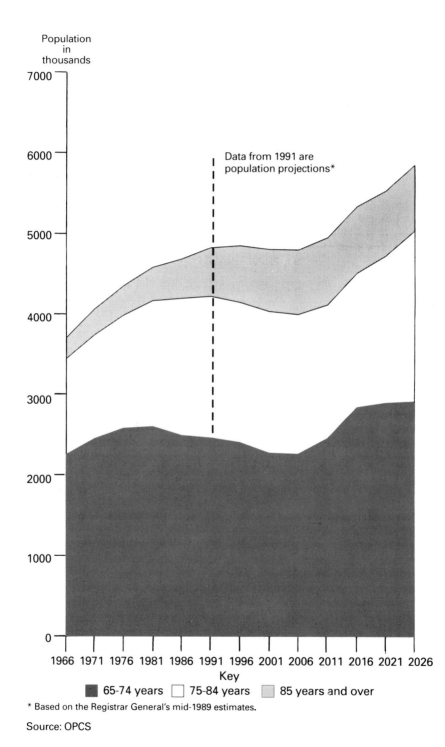

Key
65-74 years 75-84 years 85 years and over

* Based on the Registrar General's mid-1989 estimates.

Source: OPCS

Table 3.1: *Changes in household structure of people over 65 years-of-age, Great Britain, 1962-85*

	1962 %	1976 %	1980 %	1985 %
Living alone	22	30	34	36
Living with spouse only	33	44	45	45
Living with others	44	27	21	18
Total	100*	100*	100*	100*

* Total may not add up to 100 because of rounding.

Source: GHS 1980 and 1986, and Household structure of the elderly in Britain: Dale, Evadron and Arber. Ageing and Society, 1987; 37-56

An important challenge for the next decade is to ensure that the additional years of life expectancy are as free from disease and disability as possible, compressing morbidity into the final phase of life so that increased life expectancy does not lead to longer periods of ill health and dependency[3]. A second challenge will be to provide services for health promotion, prevention, treatment and care which meet the diverse needs of this changing and growing population of people in later life. Above all it will be crucial to convince older people that, by adjusting their lifestyles, they are still able to secure improvements in their quality of life and diminish the risk of illness.

Common sources of information

The GHS is a continuous survey covering a sample of all households. It includes people living in Part III accommodation, but excludes residents of long-stay hospitals and old people's homes. Results are therefore applicable only to people living at home. It is estimated that 4% of people over 65 years live in institutional care.

The OPCS surveys of disability in Great Britain were commissioned by the Department of Health and Social Security (DHSS) in 1984. They aim to provide information about the numbers of disabled people, their circumstances, and the different levels of severity. Four separate surveys were carried out between 1985 and 1988.

References

1   Office of Population Censuses and Surveys. *National population projections: mid-1989 based*. London: HMSO, 1991. (OPCS Monitor PP2 91/1).

2   Office of Population Censuses and Surveys. *General Household Survey 1986*. London: HMSO, 1989. (Series GHS no 16).

3   Kane RL, Evans JG, Macfadyen D eds. *Improving the health of older people*. Oxford: Oxford University Press, 1990.

(b) Measures of morbidity

Perceived health

Figure 3.3 shows the selected causes of long-standing illness reported by men and women aged 65-74 years and 75 years and over interviewed in the 1988 GHS[1]. Reported long-standing illnesses were higher in women at all ages, and

71

Figure 3.3: *Selected causes of self-reported long-standing illness by age-group, Great Britain, 1988*

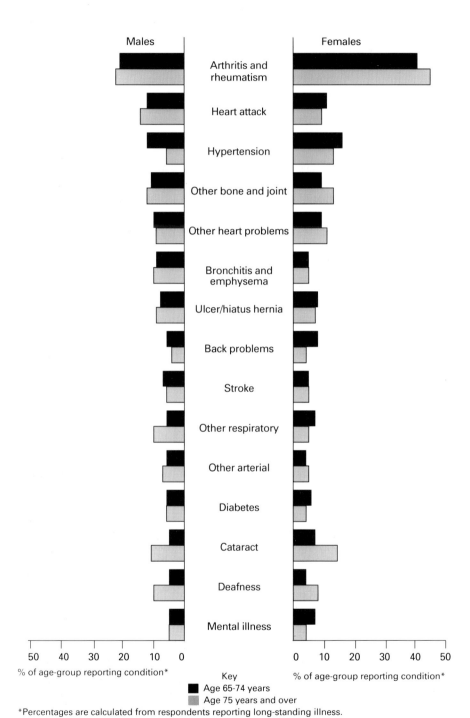

50   40   30   20   10   0   0   10   20   30   40   50

% of age-group reporting condition*   Key   % of age-group reporting condition*

■ Age 65-74 years
▨ Age 75 years and over

*Percentages are calculated from respondents reporting long-standing illness.

Source: GHS 1988 (unpublished)

increased with age in both sexes.

Figure 3.4 shows the nature of disabilities reported in the 1985 OPCS disability survey[2]. There was a high prevalence of difficulties with locomotion, hearing, sight and personal care, particularly in people aged 75 years and over. Figure 3.5 illustrates the change in the ability to perform selected self-care tasks with age, using data from the GHS.

Use of primary health care services and prescribed medicines

Figure 3.6, taken from the 3rd study of morbidity statistics from general practice[3], summarises the consultation rates in general practice for people aged 65-74 years and 75 years and over. The total consultation rates for women were higher than for men of the same age-group. The main reasons for consultations were similar in people aged 65-74 years and 75 years and over, and included diseases of the circulatory system, the respiratory system, the musculoskeletal system and the nervous system, symptoms and signs which are ill-defined, mental illness, and the category of accidents, injury, poisoning and violence.

In the 1986 GHS[4], in the month before interview 23% of people aged 75 years and over had contact with the doctor in the surgery, and 18% contact with the doctor at home. Home visits increased with age and surgery visits reduced. Contact with a chiropodist was common (11% of people); and 5% of people aged 75-79 years and 20% aged 85 years and over had contact with a district nurse.

A 1984 national survey, *Elderly People, their Medicines and their Doctors[5]*, comprised interviews with a representative sample of people aged 65 years and over, and collection of additional information from a proportion of their general practitioners (GPs). Almost 40% of people aged 65 years and over had taken no prescribed medication in the previous 24 hours, although the number of medications taken tended to increase with age. A very small percentage, approximately 5% of people aged 65 years and over, took five or more prescribed medicines. The most common categories of prescribed medicine were diuretics, hypnotics, sedatives, anxiolytics, aspirin and other analgesics (see Figure 3.7), all of which were taken more frequently in older age-groups.

There has been a rise in prescribing for people in later life in excess of that for all other groups, so that the average number of prescription items per person of pensionable age in 1990 was over three times the number per head in other age-groups. The medicines prescribed are often new and powerful. Therapeutic benefits must be balanced against the increased sensitivity of older people to medicines, and the possibility of side-effects outweighing them.

Hospital admissions

Information on the use of hospital inpatient services can be obtained from the Hospital In-patient Enquiry (HIPE)[6], which was based on a 1 in 10 sample of discharges and deaths in acute hospitals (excluding maternity and psychiatric beds). The discharge and death rate is higher for those aged 65 years and over than for any other age-group, reflecting the important impact of people in later life on the use of hospital services (see Figure 3.8). The admission rate for these

Figure 3.4: *Estimates of disablement prevalence rates by residence, disability and age-group, Great Britain, 1985*

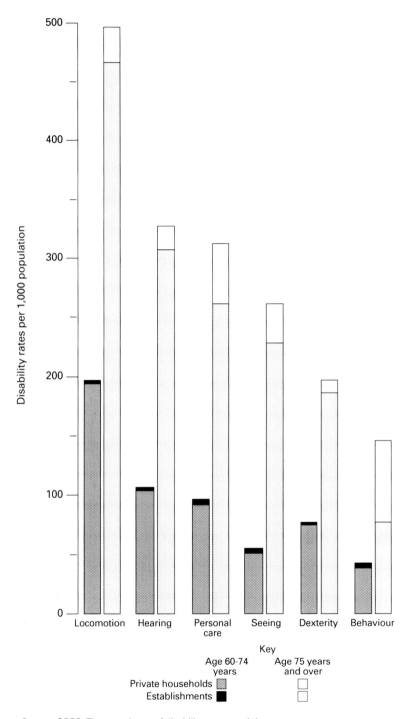

Source: OPCS. The prevalence of disability among adults

Figure 3.5: *Inability to manage selected tasks independently by sex and age-group, Great Britain, 1985*

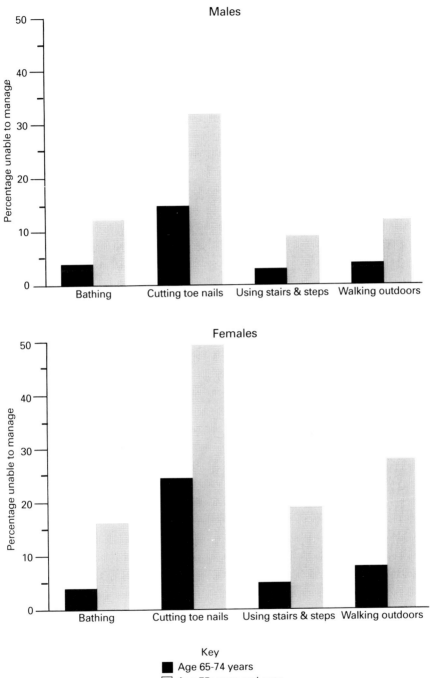

Source: GHS 1986

Figure 3.6: *Patients consulting a GP: age specific GP consultation rates by disease category, England and Wales, 1981/82*

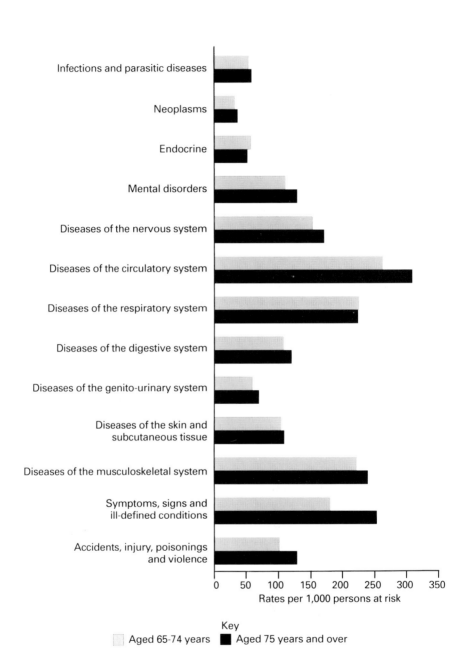

Source: OPCS Morbidity Statistics from General Practice, 1981/82

Figure 3.7: *Survey of prescribed medicines and the elderly: variations with age in the types of medicines taken, England, 1984*

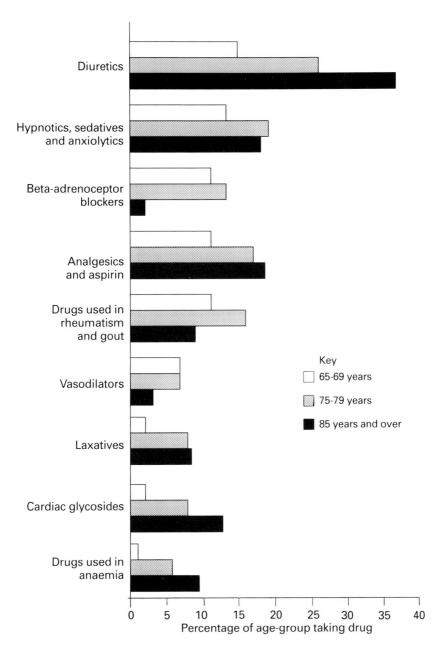

Source: Cartwright A, Smith C. Elderly people, their medicines and their doctors, 1988

Figure 3.8: *Hospital discharge (and death) rates by sex and age-group, England, 1985*

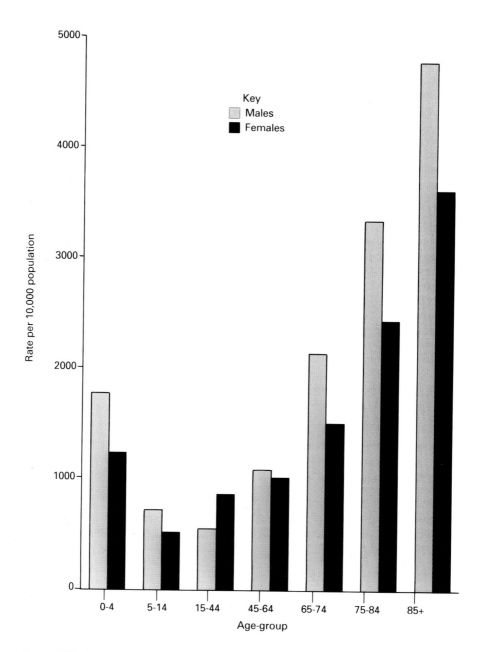

older people is higher for men than for women, a reverse of the trends found for self-reported illness or for GP consultations.

The main categories of diseases in later life for both men and women are: diseases of the circulatory system, neoplasms, diseases of the respiratory system, symptoms and signs which are ill-defined, injury and poisoning, and diseases of the digestive system, similar to the diseases which lead to general practice consultations (see Figure 3.9). It is important to remember that people aged 65 years and over are usually treated in outpatient departments and wards in acute general hospitals, rather than in specialist facilities for older people, and that after treatment most return directly to their own homes.

Cancer registrations

In men aged 65 years and over, the most frequent newly diagnosed cancer is cancer of the trachea, bronchus and lung (rate per 100,000 population increases from 439 at age 65-69 years to 652 at age 85 years and over). The rates for newly diagnosed cancer of the prostate and bladder rise with increasing age (rates per 100,000 population at age 85 years and over: 610 for cancer of the prostate (4.7 times the rate at age 65-69 years), and 250 for cancer of the bladder (2.4 times the rate at age 65-69 years)). In women, cancer of the breast is the most frequent in all older age-groups, and the rate increases slightly with age. The rates for cancer of the cervix reduce slightly with age (to 21 per 100,000 at age 85 years and over). Rates of newly diagnosed cancers of the stomach, colon, oesophagus and pancreas all increase with age, and are 2-5 times more common in people aged 85 years and over compared with people aged 65-69 years, for both men and women.

Mental health

It is difficult to estimate accurately the prevalence of mental illness in people in later life in the community. Surveys which rely on self-reported illness, such as the GHS, are likely to under-estimate prevalence due to under-reporting, and the difficulties of interviewing people with mental health problems.

Dementia

A report from the Royal College of Physicians (RCP) reviewed several studies of the prevalence of dementia. Moderate or severe dementia was found in 5-7.1% of people aged 65 years and over[7]. The incidence and prevalence of dementia increase with age, and so prevalence depends on the age-group of the population studied. The incidence of Alzheimer's disease (the most prevalent form of dementia) at the age of 80 years may be up to twentyfold that at the age of 60 years[8]. People with moderate and severe dementia may be at home, in residential homes, or in hospital, either in long-term care or being treated for another condition. In a survey of 12 Part III local authority homes, one third of residents had severe dementia, and a further third had mild to moderate dementia[9].

Depression

The prevalence of depression in people in later life has been much less

Figure 3.9: *Hospital discharge (and death) rates for selected categories by sex and age-group, England, 1985*

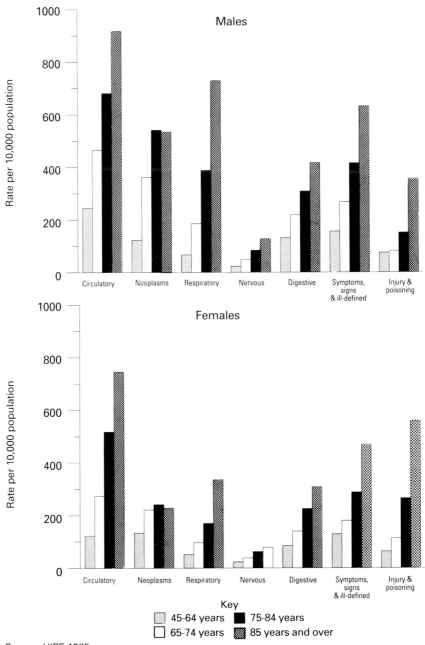

Figure 3.10: *Mental illness in the elderly: top five causes of admission by diagnostic group, sex and age-group, England, 1986*

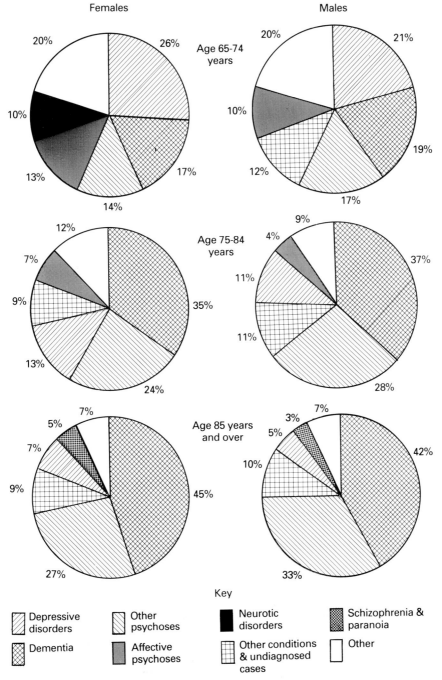

Females

Males

Age 65-74 years

Females: 26%, 17%, 14%, 13%, 10%, 20%

Males: 21%, 19%, 17%, 12%, 10%, 20%

Age 75-84 years

Females: 35%, 24%, 13%, 9%, 7%, 12%

Males: 37%, 28%, 11%, 11%, 4%, 9%

Age 85 years and over

Females: 45%, 27%, 9%, 7%, 5%, 7%

Males: 42%, 33%, 10%, 5%, 3%, 7%

Key

| Depressive disorders | Other psychoses | Neurotic disorders | Schizophrenia & paranoia |
| Dementia | Affective psychoses | Other conditions & undiagnosed cases | Other |

Percentages may not add up to 100 due to rounding.

Source: Mental Health Enquiry

81

frequently reported. Clinical depression in older people has been reported at rates of 12.9% (London, 1981), 5.2% (Liverpool, 1987), 4.3% (Nottingham, 1987) and most recently 15.9% (London, 1990), increasing to 18.5% when the residents of the local authority homes were included[10]. Depression was much commoner in people who were not currently married and in those living alone.

Admission to hospital

Figure 3.10 shows the five principal causes of admission to mental illness hospitals for men and women taken from the 1986 Mental Health Enquiry[11]. Depressive disorders were a main cause of admission in all age-groups for both men and women—ranging from 5% to 26% of all admissions; the proportion of admissions due to depressive disorders was highest in people aged 65-74 years. Senile and pre-senile dementia were more common in older age-groups, and in men and women aged 85 years and over accounted for 42% and 45% of admissions respectively. A wide range of other mental health problems was also seen.

Sensory impairment

Sight

The OPCS survey of disability in Great Britain was conducted on a sample of households and institutions. The prevalence of disability involving sight in private households was 52 per 1,000 persons aged 60-74 years and 225 per 1,000 persons aged 75 years and over. For the total population, including those in residential establishments, the prevalence was 56 per 1,000 persons aged 60-74 years, and 262 per 1,000 persons aged 75 years and over. 22% of all adults reporting disability had eye complaints; almost a quarter of these were due to cataract, but most of the remainder were not classified further[2].

The main causes of blindness and partial sight among adults admitted to local authority registers of the blind and partially sighted were last reported by age-group in 1980/81[12]. Figures for 1990/91 are currently being analysed. 76% of the registered blind population are aged 65 years and over, and 59% are aged 75 years and over. Data from the registers showed that degeneration of the macula and posterior pole was responsible for over 40% of cases of blindness in people aged 65 years. Only three other conditions accounted for more than 5%—open-angle glaucoma, senile cataract and diabetic retinopathy. The importance of degeneration of the macula and posterior pole as a cause of blindness in all elderly persons increased markedly with ageing, from 28% in the 65-74 years age-group to 52% in those aged 85 years and over. On the other hand, diabetic retinopathy and myopia became less frequent.

The figures reported from registration are likely to represent a considerable underestimation of severity. Of people who satisfy the criteria to register as blind, a considerable proportion choose not to register, and of those who register quite a number of forms go astray and are not received for analysis. A revised version of Form BD8, completed by ophthalmologists to certify blindness and partial sight, was introduced on 1 April 1990. The form is used for registering a person as visually impaired with the Social Services Department where he or she resides. The revised form includes provision for the blind person to give consent to the disclosure of information to named third parties, and copies of the form are provided for the patient and the GP, as well as for the local Social Services Department. There is also an epidemiological return, giving the causes of blindness or partial sight, for OPCS.

A study of eye disease in a randomly selected age-stratified sample of people aged 76 years and over in Melton Mowbray was conducted by an ophthalmologist to determine the prevalence of major sight-threatening conditions. Senile cataract was found in 46.1% of people, senile macular degeneration in 41.5%, and open-angle glaucoma in 6.6%[13]. The figures are considerably higher than those found by self-reporting in the OPCS survey or by registration.

Hearing

The 1986 GHS[4] found that over 35% of men and over 29% of women aged 65 years and over had difficulty with hearing. The proportion with hearing problems increased with age (see Figure 3.11), but in all age-groups less than half (as low as one fifth in men aged 65-69 years) of those with difficulty in hearing wore a hearing aid.

The Medical Research Council (MRC) Institute of Hearing Research in Nottingham reported much higher prevalences of hearing disabilities[14]. The first stage of its study analysed the responses to a postal questionnaire from a random sample of people on the electoral registers of four cities—Nottingham, Cardiff, Glasgow and Southampton. 35% of people aged 61-70 years, 44% of those aged 71-80 years, and 60% of those aged 81 years and over reported great difficulty hearing speech in noisy surroundings. Prolonged spontaneous tinnitus was reported by 16% of people aged 61-70 years and 14% of those aged 71-80 years. In the second stage of the study, a random sample of people returning questionnaires was offered audiological assessment. Over one third (37%) of people aged 61-70 years and 60% of people aged 71-80 years had at least mild impairment (categorised as a decibel hearing threshold level (dBHL) of greater than or equal to 25) in both ears; calculation of the level was based on the hearing in the better ear. 7% of people aged 61-70 years and 18% of those aged 71-80 years had at least moderate impairment in both ears.

References

1   Office of Population Censuses and Surveys. *General Household Survey 1988*. London: HMSO, 1990. (Series GHS no 19)

2   Office of Population Censuses and Surveys. *The prevalence of disability among adults*. London: HMSO, 1988. (OPCS surveys of disability in Great Britain; report 1).

3   Royal College of General Practitioners, Office of Population Censuses and Surveys, Department of Health and Social Security. *Morbidity statistics from general practice: third national survey 1981-1982*. London: HMSO, 1986.

4   Office of Population Censuses and Surveys. *General Household Survey 1986*. London: HMSO, 1989. (Series GHS no 16).

5   Cartwright A, Smith C. *Elderly people, their medicines and their doctors*. London: Routledge, 1988.

6   Department of Health and Social Security. *Hospital In-patient Enquiry (HIPE)*. London: Department of Health and Social Security, 1985.

7   Royal College of Physicians: Committee on Geriatrics. Organic Mental Impairment in the elderly: implications for research, education and the provision of services. *JR Coll Physicians Lond* 1981; **15**(3).

8   Katzman N. *Alzheimer's disease as an age-dependent disorder*. In: Fogarty JE, ed. Research and the ageing population. Chichester: Wiley, 1988; 69-80. (CIBA Foundation Symposium; 134).

9   Mann A, Graham N, Ashby D. Psychiatric illness in residential homes for the elderly: a survey in one London Borough. *Age Ageing* 1984; **13**: 257-65.

Figure 3.11: *Difficulty with hearing in the elderly by sex and age-group, Great Britain, 1985*

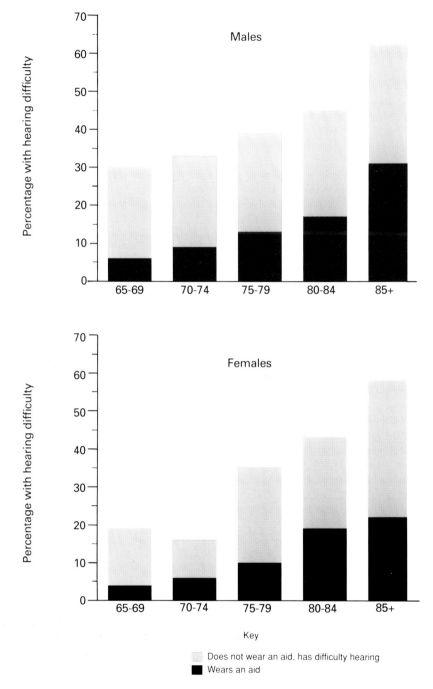

Key
Does not wear an aid. has difficulty hearing
Wears an aid

Source: GHS 1986

84

10 Livingstone G, Hawkins A, Graham N, Blizard B, Mann AH. The Gospel Oak Study: Prevalence rates of dementia, depression and activity limitation among elderly residents in Inner London. *Psychol Med* 1990; **20**: 137-46.

11 Department of Health and Social Security. *Mental health statistics for England: 1986*. London: Department of Health and Social Security, 1987.

12 Department of Health and Social Security. *Causes of blindness and partial sight among adults in 1976/77 and 1980/81: England*. London: HMSO, 1988.

13 Gibson JM, Rosenthal AR, Lavery J. A study of the prevalence of eye disease in the elderly in an English community. *Trans Ophthalmol Soc UK* 1985; **104**: 196-203.

14 Davis AC. The prevalence of hearing impairment and reported hearing disability among adults in Great Britain. *Int J Epidemiol* 1989; **4**: 911-7.

(c) Social circumstances and care

People in later life are more likely than younger people to own their home outright, although older people living alone include the highest proportion of any group renting accommodation privately or from the council (see Table 3.2). People in later life who live alone are less likely than younger people to have a telephone. However, the 1988 Family Expenditure Survey[1] demonstrated that, in both single-person and two-person households, the income distribution of retired people is concentrated at the lower end of the income range compared with that of people who have not retired. In particular, for single incomes of less than £80 per week, and dual incomes of less than £125 a week, pensioners form the major category. The 1988 Family Expenditure Survey also showed that average weekly expenditure was less in households where the head was aged 75 years or more (£99), and in those with heads of households aged 65-74 years (£138), than in households with younger heads aged 50-64 years (£223). The proportion of income spent on personal and household services and fuel increased with age, whereas expenditure on food and transport costs declined.

The 1986 GHS reported on the unaccompanied use of public transport by people aged 65 years and over. There were 74% of women and 55% of men aged 65-69 years who could use public transport, but use fell with age, especially for women, and in those aged 85 years and over 52% of men and only 19% of women were able to use public transport unaccompanied. The main reasons given by non-users were car ownership (or access to another car) and ill health or disability. Ill health or disability was a reason given more by those who were female, older and living alone. Overall, of those aged 65 years or more who did not have a car, 28% did not use public transport.

Age-related contact with personal social services is summarised in Figure 3.12, which shows that contact with all agencies increased with age; in the month before interview 36% of people aged 85 years and over had contact with a home help, and 11% had contact with meals on wheels. Additional information on contact with services is available from the OPCS disability surveys, which show that the proportion of adults receiving services increases with disability and age. In the survey of private households, 30% of the most severely disabled adults aged 75 years and over received home help services. Of all disabled adults aged 75 years and over, 18% thought they needed additional domiciliary services, compared with 14% of those aged 65-74 years[2].

Residential care

Between 1977 and 1987 the number of residents aged 65 years and over in local

Figure 3.12: *Contact with selected personal social services in the month before interview by age-group, Great Britain, 1985*

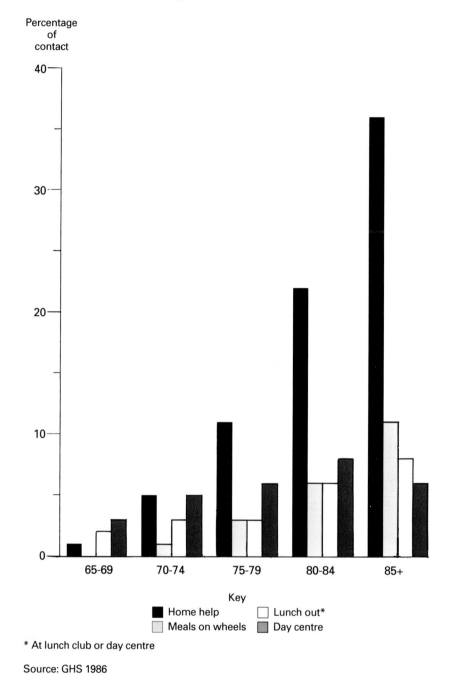

Percentage
of
contact

Key
■ Home help   □ Lunch out*
▨ Meals on wheels   ▨ Day centre

* At lunch club or day centre

Source: GHS 1986

Table 3.2: *Housing tenure and amenities for elderly people, Great Britain, 1985*

	Elderly person living with spouse only	Elderly person living alone	Elderly person in other kinds of household	Households containing no elderly persons
	%	%	%	%
Tenure:				
Owner occupied, owned outright	55	40	43	15
Owner occupied, with mortgage	4	1	15	50
Rented from local authority or New Town	33	47	34	27
Rented privately	8	12	8	9
Availability of w/c	99	97	98	99
Availability of bath/shower	99	97	98	100
Central heating	68	59	62	72
Car ownership	56	12	58	72
Telephone	87	69	80	83

Source: GHS 1986

authority and voluntary homes remained much the same. In 1977 there were 101,681 residents in local authority homes and 24,284 residents in voluntary homes. The corresponding figures for 1987 were 100,594 and 25,068. The number of residents in private homes increased by a factor of 3.7, from 22,920 in 1977 to 84,852 in 1987[3]. However, the number of residents aged 65 years and over in homes where local authorities were contributing to the individual's cost fell between 1979 and 1989, from 102,086 to 94,224 in local authority homes, 12,886 to 2,205 in voluntary homes, and 2,164 to 702 in private homes.

References

1 Central Statistical Office. *Family expenditure survey 1988*. London: HMSO, 1990.

2 Office of Population Censuses and Surveys. *Disabled adults: services, transport and employment*. London: HMSO, 1989. (OPCS surveys of disability in Great Britain; report 4).

3 Department of Health. *Health and personal social services statistics for England. 1989 edition*. London: HMSO, 1989.

(d) Palliative care

The last decade has witnessed rapid growth of the modern hospice movement, and Ministers have announced that an additional £17 million will be made available in 1991/92 to supplement health authorities' existing support. The majority of people who die are aged 65 years and over. In a national survey based on a random sample of 639 adult (aged 15 years or more) deaths registered in England, interviewers tried to contact the person who could tell them most about the last 12 months in the lives of the deceased people[1]. 23% of the people who died were aged 65-74 years, 32% 75-84 years and 23% 85 years and over. 4% of people had received some form of hospice care, but, although people who died in hospices had better pain relief, there was no indication of any dissemination of hospice practice to other services in the areas around hospices. Thus, a major challenge for the 1990s is to extend the principles of good palliative care to the treatment of all patients with a terminal illness, regardless of their underlying diagnosis, and to measure the effectiveness of care in these settings[2].

References

1   Cartwright A, Seale C. *The natural history of a survey*. London: King Edward's Hospital Fund for London, 1990.
2   Higginson IJ, McCarthy M. Evaluation of palliative care: steps to quality assurance. *Palliative Medicine* 1989; **3**: 267-74.

(e) Carers of older people

The increasing emphasis on community-based programmes for the care of elderly and infirm sufferers[1] depends to a large extent on the mobilisation and maintenance of informal support systems. Most elderly people who need assistance with either personal or domestic tasks rely on relatives to provide it[2]. Estimates of the replacement cost of all informal care lie between £15 and £24 billion per annum[3]. This figure is likely to continue to rise as the number of people aged 65 years and over increases, and the emphasis on community care, outlined in the White Paper *Caring for People*[1], takes effect. A carer may be involved in dealing with practical and behavioural problems, in addition to a change in lifestyle, and this can lead to physical and mental health problems in the carer.

The 1985 GHS[4] included a series of questions to identify people looking after a sick, handicapped or elderly person. One adult in seven (14%) was providing informal care, and one in five households (19%) contained a carer. One adult carer in five was aged 65 years and over. A small survey by the National Consumer Council of carers of elderly people with dementia living at home identified the following areas of need: early diagnosis; information and advice, especially in the early stages; counselling; the availability of a sitting service; information about possible residential care (for long-term planning); and a prompt, reliable ambulance service to day care or respite care[5].

References

1   Department of Health. *Caring for People: community care in the next decade and beyond*. London: HMSO, 1990. (Cm. 849).
2   Bowling A. *The health and social service needs of people aged 85+ living at home*. London: City and Hackney Health Authority, 1988.
3   Family policy studies centre. *Family Policy Bulletin 6*. London: Family policy studies centre, 1989.
4   Green H. *Informal Carers: a study carried out on behalf of the Department of Health and Social Security as part of the 1985 General Household Survey*. London: HMSO, 1988.
5   National Consumer Council. *Consulting consumers in the NHS: services for people with dementia living at home*. London: National Consumer Council, 1990.

(f) Health promotion

Maintaining health

Some information on the behaviour of older people which is likely to influence their health is available from the 1986 GHS[1]. 29% of men and 22% of women aged 60 years and over smoked. 13% of men in this age range were drinking more than the 'sensible drinking' limit of 21 units of alcohol per week, and 3% of women more than the limit of 14 units per week. The same survey showed that only 31% of men and 22% of women aged 65-74 years, and 20% of men and 9% of women aged 75 years and over, took exercise in the four weeks before the survey.

A recent WHO publication, *Improving the Health of Older People*[2], included recommendations on the following topics:

Prudent diet—sufficient to maintain normal weight and avoid obesity, including plenty of vegetables, fruits and calcium-containing foods (preferably milk products), but restricting fat and salt. Further education in the choice of desirable foods and guidance on the selection of prepared convenience foods is needed. A Department of Health (DH) working group on nutrition in older people is due to report in 1992.

Weight control—underweight or overweight present health risks. Gross overweight limits mobility, strains cardiac function, and increases the risk of hypertension, diabetes and premature death. Those very much above the desirable weight should make efforts to lose weight by diet and exercise.

In contrast, in some frail elderly people, particularly those living in institutions, appetite may be so poor that food intake may be sufficient to maintain body weight. In these circumstances efforts should be made to encourage sufficient food intake to reach and maintain a sensible weight.

Exercise—the habit of regularly taking exercise should be started earlier in life, and should be continued as long as possible for its beneficial effects on self-esteem, mobility, cardiovascular function, osteoporosis, and longevity. Benefits are found even when exercise is started late in life.

Smoking cigarettes—harmful at any age. Even over the age of 70 years, continued smoking is a risk factor for heart and respiratory disease and for osteoporosis. Diseases of the circulatory system are a major cause of morbidity and the main cause of mortality (see Table 3.3) in older people, and there is good evidence that stopping smoking, even late in life, reduces that risk.

Social life and social contacts—improve the quality of life and stimulate mental and physical activity. The kinds of activity where older people meet others of all ages, and engage in pleasurable and educational activities, can provide peer pressure and support for changes in behaviour which are aimed at promoting health.

The same risk factors for heart disease and stroke as operate in middle age, such as hypertension, smoking and blood lipids, continue to operate in old age. The European study of the treatment of hypertension in the elderly demonstrated differences in cardiovascular mortality between treated and untreated groups of hypertensives aged 60 years and over[3]. Benefits were demonstrated up to the age of 80 years. An RCP Working Party on Cardiological Intervention on Elderly People has been meeting during 1990 and is due to report in 1991.

Table 3.3: *Main causes of mortality by ICD Group, England and Wales, 1988*

| Causes | Numbers and percentages* Age-group (years) | | | | | |
	65-74	(%)	75-84	(%)	85+	(%)
Males						
Diseases of the circulatory system	39827	(49)	46392	(49)	15580	(46)
Diseases of the respiratory system	7579	(9)	12927	(14)	6858	(20)
Neoplasms	25823	(32)	23605	(25)	5561	(16)
Other causes	7641	(9)	12382	(13)	5949	(18)
All causes	80870	(100)	95306	(100)	33948	(100)
Females						
Diseases of the circulatory system	25601	(45)	55810	(54)	46297	(53)
Diseases of the respiratory system	4388	(8)	9358	(9)	13172	(15)
Neoplasms	19040	(34)	20951	(20)	9508	(11)
Other causes	7538	(13)	17547	(17)	18259	(21)
All causes	56567	(100)	103666	(100)	87236	(100)

* Totals may not add up to 100 due to rounding.

Sources: OPCS Mortality Statistics

The 4th Winter Warmth Campaign, *Keep Warm, Keep Well*, was launched in 1990. As with the first three, Government Departments (Health, Social Security, Environment and Energy) and voluntary bodies (Age Concern, Help the Aged and Neighbourhood Energy Action) united to help vulnerable and older people keep warm and healthy during cold weather. The purpose of the campaign was to inform and educate people at risk from the cold weather to take steps to minimise the risks, and to advise them of what help was available. The main thrust of the campaign provided information based on simple preventive measures that people could take for themselves, such as clothing, diet and exercise. It also covered a wide range of available help and services, and advice on benefits, home insulation, draught proofing, efficient use of heating, and budgeting for fuel costs.

The information was available to the public:

- As a booklet available in English, Welsh, Bengali, Gujerati, Hindi, Punjabi, Urdu, Chinese, Greek, Polish and Turkish.

- On the Winter Warmth Line, a free '0800' telephone number run by Help the Aged.

- As an audio cassette recording of the booklet for the visually impaired.

– In TV and radio 'fillers'.

The total cost of the 1989/90 campaign was £440,000.

Preventing accidents

Until 1977, there was little national evidence about accidents and falls. The Home Accident Surveillance System was established to collect data on a sample of hospital casualty attendances, and provide some information on the nature of accidents in the elderly. Accidents and accidental deaths, of which fractures are the single major cause, increase with age. Location of accident is available for only 50% of all recorded cases, but this shows an increasing proportion of accidents occurring within the home as age increases.

Statistics from the Home Accident Deaths Database indicate that over 70% of all fatal accidents in the home in England and Wales were to people aged over 65 years. It is estimated, in the 12th Annual Report of the Home Accident Surveillance System, that some 304,000 people aged 65 years and over attend a hospital Accident and Emergency Department each year in England and Wales as a result of a home accident[4].

In people aged 65-74 years, 34% of home accidents where the location in the home is known occur in the kitchen or garden, whereas for people aged 75 years and over the living/dining room is the most common place for an accident (19%), followed by the bedroom (18%) and the kitchen (14%). Falls were the major cause of home accidents, comprising 65.3% of all accidents for which hospital treatment was sought by people aged 65 years and over[4].

Approximately one third of all people aged 65 years and over experience one or more falls a year; people living in institutions are generally more likely to fall than those living in the community. Women and older elderly people are more likely to fall than men or younger elderly people. Identifying the cause is difficult. There is a multiplicity of factors; medical problems play an important part, particularly among very elderly people. Disability, disturbances of gait, vision, and hand-grip strength, and specific or non-specific ill health (such as disorders of the cardiovascular or neurological systems) can all be implicated. Environmental hazards, for example steps, stairs or badly placed or unstable furnishings and fittings, are also known to contribute[5].

There are very few studies assessing the effectiveness of programmes to prevent home accidents. *A Review of Research on Falls Among Elderly People*[5], published in 1990, examined the studies to date and recommended the following preventive strategies:

– Heightening the awareness of everyone to the dangers of falls to elderly people.

– Educating professionals, such as architects, planners and health visitors, to think constantly about safety in general, and falls in particular, and to develop strategies which successfully reduce the number of falls.

- Educating elderly people and their carers to recognise potential risk situations, to take action which avoids them, and to know what to do if a fall occurs.

- Targeting programmes to high-risk groups.

- Creating check lists of risk areas for elderly people, their carers and professionals.

Preventing and detecting disease

In the White Paper *Promoting Better Health*[6], the Government declared its intention to introduce, through changes in the remuneration system, encouragement for GPs to provide comprehensive regular care for elderly people. The new contract for GPs, which was introduced on 1 April 1990, includes a requirement to offer health promotion and disease prevention advice to all patients, and in particular a requirement for an assessment to be offered annually to all patients over the age of 75 years, and for a similar check to be offered every three years to patients between the ages of 16 and 74 years.

An annual assessment of sensory functions, mobility, mental condition, physical condition (including incontinence), social environment and the use of medicines, and the offer of a home visit, are included in the contract. They should help the early detection of disease and disability, improve the quality of life and maintain social functioning, which is the prime objective of the care of old people. The MRC is starting a strong initiative to develop research into the most effective way of carrying out this surveillance.

Preventing and detecting mental illness

Although depressed individuals are more than usually likely to have been in contact with their GP and local hospital in the previous month, antidepressant medication seems to be infrequently prescribed[7], even though its effectiveness in treating depression in older people is well described[8]. This suggests a need for further education and training of primary health care staff in the detection and management of depression, as depression seriously restricts quality of life and can lead to suicide.

There may be opportunities for the prevention of dementia caused by cerebrovascular disease, although research is needed to demonstrate the effectiveness of prevention and intervention programmes. However, the current management of people with dementia relies on the appropriate and effective combined delivery of health and supportive social services.

Services for mentally ill older people are provided in many settings. The Health Advisory Service is an independent service aiming to help to maintain and improve standards of management and organisation of patient care, through a rolling programme of visits to health Districts by multidisciplinary teams. Its remit includes services for elderly people. Reports during 1990, as well as praising the dedication of staff and highlighting areas of good practice, identified problems in many Districts with joint planning and working, lack of a clearly stated policy and inadequate respite services.

Continence

The prevalence of urinary incontinence is estimated to be between 7% and 11% in people aged 65 years and over, considerably higher than the reported provision of personal incontinence aids by the National Health Service (NHS)[9,10]. In 1988, DH issued a Health Notice advising health authorities to develop a continence advisory service which should include a continence adviser, a doctor with a special responsibility for incontinence services, access to urodynamic services if appropriate, and physiotherapy[11]. It is probable that patients' failure to communicate the problem to the primary health care team, often because of embarrassment, has contributed to poor management of an often deeply distressing problem. The annual health check by the primary health care team provides an opportunity for enquiries to be made about the presence of incontinence, and, where appropriate, to arrange referral to the continence advisory service for expert assessment and appropriate treatment.

References

1 Office of Population Censuses and Surveys. *General Household Survey 1986*. London: HMSO, 1989. (Series GHS no16).

2 Kane RL, Evans JG, Macfadyen D eds. *Improving the health of older people*. Oxford: Oxford University Press, 1990.

3 Amery A, Brixxo R, Clement D et al. Efficacy of antihypertensive drug treatment according to age, sex, blood pressure and previous cardiovascular disease in patients over the age of 60. *Lancet* 1986; **ii**: 589-92.

4 Department of Trade and Industry. *Home and leisure accidents report*. London: Department of Trade and Industry, 1988.

5 Age Concern Institute of Gerontology. *A review of research on falls among elderly people*. London: Department of Trade and Industry, 1990.

6 Department of Health and Social Security. *Promoting Better Health; the Government's programme for improving primary health care*. London: HMSO, 1987. (Cm. 249).

7 Livingstone G, Hawkins A, Graham N, Blizard B, Mann AH. The Gospel Oak Study: prevalence rates of dementia, depression and activity limitation among elderly residents in Inner London. *Psychol Med* 1990; **20**: 137-46.

8 Gurland BJ, Mayeux R, Meyers BS. *The effectiveness of intervention for the mental health of the elderly*. In: Kane RL, Evans JG, Macfadyen D, eds. Improving the health of older people: a world review. Oxford: Oxford University Press, 1990; 262-72.

9 McGrother CW, Carleden C, Duffin H, Clarke M. A profile of disordered micturition in the elderly at home. *Age Ageing* 1987; **16**: 105-10.

10 Thomas TM, Plymat KR, Blannin J, Meade TW. Prevalence of urinary incontinence. *Br Med J* 1980; **281**: 1243-5.

11 Department of Health. *Health service development: the development of services for people with physical or sensory disabilities*. Heywood (Lancashire): Department of Health, 1988. (Health Notice: HN(88)26).

(g) Rehabilitation

Ensuring that older people spend the minimum time necessary in hospital has created substantial pressures on rehabilitation services. Many elderly people have multiple problems and are very frail, and need rehabilitation in the community as well as in hospital. While there has been an encouraging increase in rehabilitation based on the patient's home, this is by no means comprehensive; too many people are still not being assisted to return to their optimum level of function. This is clearly an issue that needs to be addressed with some urgency. The success of community care policy will depend to a large extent on the outcome of rehabilitation in enabling individuals to maximise their independence, and reduce as much as possible their reliance on carers and statutory services.

The growing practice of rehabilitation staff, such as physiotherapists, occupational therapists and speech therapists, providing their services in non-traditional localities, such as GP practices and residential care establishments, is a welcome development; however, formal evaluation is still required. Collaboration of this nature is an explicit requirement of the community care arrangements, and will need to feature in community care plans.

It is encouraging to note the widespread development of skill-sharing. Professionally qualified staff have been devoting time to enhancing the skills of others, such as support staff and informal carers, enabling them to take on duties that do not need the intervention of highly qualified professionals. This has the dual benefit of improving the level of care given by every staff member who has contact with patients, and reducing costly overlaps.

Conclusion

The number of men and women living to later life has continued to increase throughout the last one hundred years; the number of people aged 85 years and over is projected to increase by 35% in the next decade.

Many of the diseases affecting people in later life are similar to those affecting people of middle age (cardiovascular diseases, respiratory diseases, cancers, mental health problems), although some diseases become much more prevalent, for example musculoskeletal problems, fracture of the femur, the dementias, depression, stroke, incontinence and certain cancers. For diseases where cure is not possible, services must be geared to the reduction of morbidity, rehabilitation and supportive care, bearing in mind that older people often have two or more health problems. The correct mix of services to meet the needs of this growing and diverse population requires development.

A major challenge for the 1990s is to develop appropriate and effective strategies to ensure that this added life is lived at a high quality, and that morbidity is compressed through appropriate and effective health promotion, disease prevention, treatment, care and rehabilitation. Effective health promotion will require collaboration between the many agencies which can influence the diet, exercise habits, lifestyle, social contacts and environment of older people. Cost-effective methods of preventing morbidity, rather than just mortality, need to be actively sought and tested. Until now, much prevention research has excluded people aged over 65 years. In the future, the effect of preventive strategies for older people will need to be considered.

Even with the most effective health promotion and disease prevention, older people will still become ill and need medical care. The organisation of secondary health care for older people is very varied[1,2,3,4], and the relationship between primary and secondary health care services is often ill-defined. It is necessary to ensure that services are organised in a way that will provide the most effective response to the developing demographic pressures.

References

1   NAHA research paper. *Will you still love me? New opportunities for health services for elderly people in the 1990s and beyond.* London: NAHA, 1989.

2   Brocklehurst JC, Lane N, Moore-Smith B. Interface between geriatric and general medicine. *Health Trends* 1989; **21**: 48-50.

3   Young A. There is no such thing as geriatric medicine, and its here to stay. *Lancet* 1989; **ii**: 263-5.

4   Acheson ED. The impending crisis of old age: a challenge to ingenuity. *Lancet* 1982; **ii**: 592-4.

4. NEEDS, EFFECTIVENESS AND OUTCOMES

Introduction

During 1990, District Health Authorities (DHAs) and Family Health Services Authorities (FHSAs) prepared themselves to purchase health care on behalf of their resident populations. Their purchasing decisions will be influenced increasingly by assessment of which interventions are effective in improving health and by the needs of their resident populations.

This chapter describes the work that the Department of Health (DH) has carried out, or commissioned, to assist authorities in their purchasing role, and developments to facilitate the monitoring and evaluation of their decisions. Part of the work involved the National Health Service (NHS) Management Executive, in association with the East Anglian Regional Health Authority, Cambridge University and the Cambridge DHA, commissioning and carrying out studies on diabetes mellitus; they are used to illustrate the principles described.

The chapter concludes with an account of the Department's initiative on developing outcome indicators for mental health care.

(a) Assessing health care needs

As described in the Report for 1989[1], authorities purchasing health care on behalf of their resident population will be responsible for the assessment of health care needs. Need for a particular package of health care depends on:

   i.   How many people have a particular problem, both in terms of the number becoming ill each year (incidence) and in terms of the number remaining ill at any one time (prevalence).

   ii.   How effective the care is (does it produce an improvement in health and well-being?).

Purchasers of health care will also obtain a perspective of what services they might purchase by:

   – seeking the views of the population, general practitioners (GPs) and other providers of health care; and

   – comparing health care provision locally with that in other DHAs and FHSAs.

The NHS Management Executive's project, 'The Role of the District Health Authority', commissioned experts to review what is known about the incidence and prevalence of particular conditions, and about the effectiveness of care for each condition reviewed. These summaries are intended to assist DHAs with their purchasing decisions; the review on diabetes mellitus illustrates the concept.

Incidence and prevalence of diabetes mellitus

There are three main forms of diabetes mellitus:

- Insulin-dependent diabetes mellitus.

- Non-insulin-dependent diabetes mellitus.

- Gestational diabetes (diabetes of pregnancy).

The prevalence of clinically diagnosed diabetes is estimated to be about 1% of the total population at any one time[2], ie approximately half a million people in England have been clinically diagnosed as having diabetes[3]. The prevalence is considerably higher for certain groups of the population—diabetes particularly affects people of Asian[4] and Afro-Caribbean origin[5]. In those of Asian origin, the prevalence of non-insulin-dependent diabetes is nearly five times that in the comparable European population. In the population as a whole the number of diagnosed diabetics may be only half the total number of diabetics[4,6,7], and, because the number increases with age, the prevalence is expected to rise over the next decade as the population ages further. It is estimated that the number of people over 70 years-of-age with clinically diagnosed diabetes will increase by about 19,000 during this period. In addition, a recent increase in the incidence of insulin-dependent diabetes in young children will result in more people with the complications of diabetes in later life (see below).

There has been an apparent slight rise in the death rate from diabetes mellitus in most age-groups, and most noticeably in the 55-74 years age-group, since the early 1980s, as shown in Figure 4.1, although changes in the coding rules for death certification, introduced in 1984, may account for much of it. The Regional variation in deaths due to diabetes is shown in Figure 4.2. In 1989, the standardised mortality ratio was highest in the West Midlands, perhaps due to the higher prevalence of non-insulin-dependent diabetes mellitus in people of Asian origin. There is a marked social class gradient in mortality due to diabetes, the rates being highest in Social Classes IV and V. The gradient between manual and non-manual groups of men of working age appears to have widened during the 1970s, as shown in Figure 4.3. England compares favourably with many other countries, although these—and other—mortality data have to be interpreted with considerable caution because of differing certification and coding practices (see Figures 4.4 and 4.5).

The main complications of diabetes are cardiovascular disease, peripheral vascular disease, nephropathy, visual impairment and neuropathy. People with diabetes are at a greatly increased risk of death from coronary artery disease and cerebrovascular disease. About 0.1% of known diabetics are likely to develop end-stage renal failure[8], and about 2% are likely to have difficulty in seeing as a result of diabetic retinopathy, although this can be prevented[9]. The commonest problem arising from diabetic neuropathy is reduced sensation in the feet, which can rapidly lead to ulceration and infection. Peripheral vascular disease is aggravated by smoking and may lead to gangrene and amputation of the lower limb.

The prevalence and impact of diabetes in an average District with a population of 250,000 is illustrated in Table 4.1.

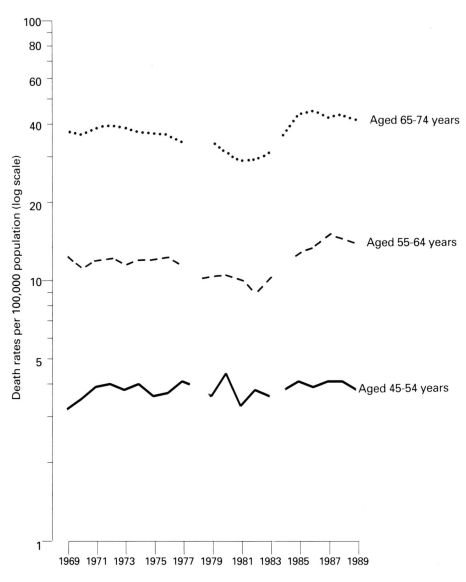

Figure 4.1: *Trends in death rates for diabetes mellitus by age-group, England, 1969-89**

*Discontinuity between 1983 and 1984 due to introduction of coding the underlying cause of death from Part II of the Death Certificate (WHO Rule 3).
Discontinuity between 1978 and 1979 due to the change from ICD 8 coding to ICD 9.

Source: OPCS

Figure 4.2: *Standardised mortality ratios for diabetes mellitus by Regional Health Authority, 1989*

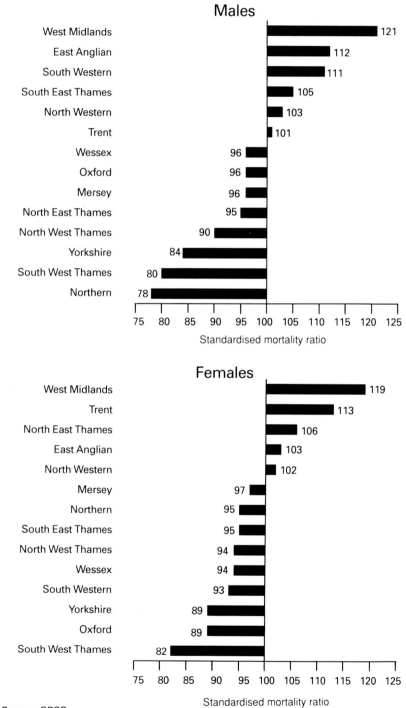

Figure 4.3: *Standardised mortality ratios for diabetes mellitus in males by social class, England and Wales, 1970-72 and 1979-83*

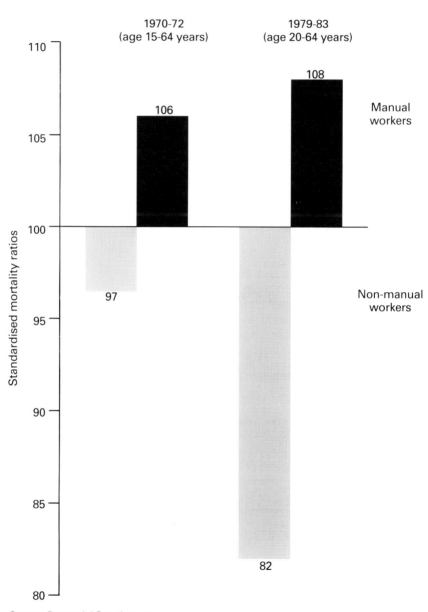

Source: Decennial Supplements

Figure 4.4: *International trends in death rates for diabetes mellitus in males aged 55-64 years, 1988**

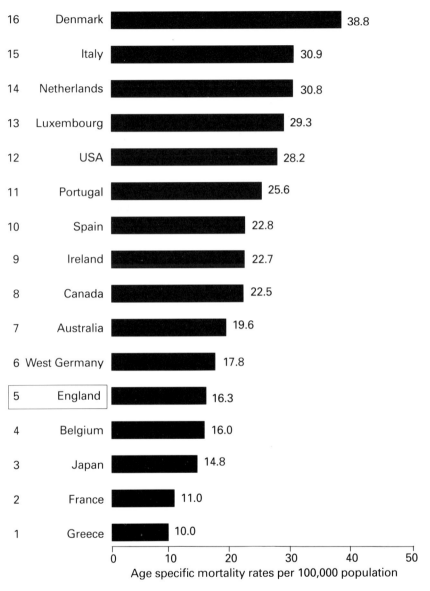

16	Denmark	38.8
15	Italy	30.9
14	Netherlands	30.8
13	Luxembourg	29.3
12	USA	28.2
11	Portugal	25.6
10	Spain	22.8
9	Ireland	22.7
8	Canada	22.5
7	Australia	19.6
6	West Germany	17.8
5	England	16.3
4	Belgium	16.0
3	Japan	14.8
2	France	11.0
1	Greece	10.0

Age specific mortality rates per 100,000 population

*Data for 1988 except for Australia, Netherlands, USA, Ireland, Denmark and France 1987, Italy and Greece 1986, and Spain 1985.

Sources: OPCS and WHO Annuals

Figure 4.5: *International trends in death rates for diabetes mellitus in females aged 55-64 years, 1988**

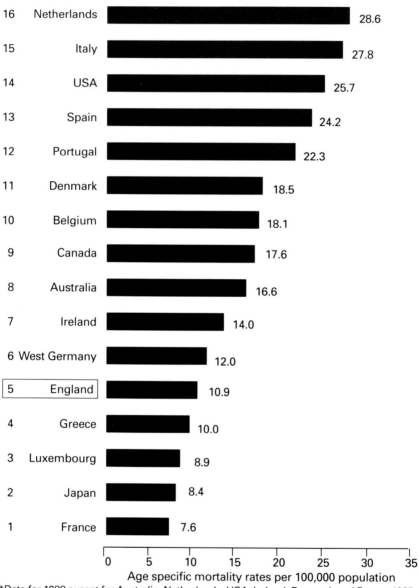

Age specific mortality rates per 100,000 population

*Data for 1988 except for Australia, Netherlands, USA, Ireland, Denmark and France 1987, Italy and Greece 1986, and Spain 1985.

Sources: OPCS and WHO Annuals

Table 4.1: *Diabetes mellitus—prevalence, health service usage, complications and mortality. Estimated numbers for District with resident population of 250,000*

Age-groups		0-14 years	15-44 years	45-64 years	65+ years	All ages
1	Population	47000	110000	54000	39000	250000
2	Estimated number of people with diabetes mellitus					
	Male	23	239	616	692	1570
	Female	16	195	353	997	1561
	Total	39	434	969	1689	3131
3	Number of people consulting GP with a diagnosis of diabetes mellitus	33	300	630	944	1907
4	Number of discharges from hospital attributed to diabetes mellitus	16	49	62	115	242
4	Average number of beds occupied daily by people with a diagnosis of diabetes mellitus	1.5% of District hospital beds				
5,6	Estimated number of people with diabetic complications					
	Cataract	12		30	175	217
	Maculopathy			20	50	70
	Complex retinopathy	35		40	130	205
	Diabetic neuropathy		255		215	470
	Foot ulcers		30		85	115
7	Estimated annual number of deaths directly attributed to diabetes mellitus			5	35	40

Sources:
1. OPCS Population Estimate, England 1989
2. Williams DRR. Hospital Admissions of Diabetic Patients: Information from Hospital Activity Analysis. Diabetic Med 1985; **2**: 27-32
3. Morbidity Statistics from General Practice 1981/82
4. Hospital Inpatient Enquiry 1985
5. Houston A. Retinopathy in the Poole Area: An Epidemiological Inquiry. Advances in diabetes epidemiology. INSERM Symposium No 22 (1982)
6. Neil HAW, Thompson QV, Thorgood M et al. Diabetes in the Elderly: The Oxford Community Diabetes Study. Diabetic Med (1989); **6**: 608-13
7. OPCS DH2 1989

References

1 Department of Health. *On the State of Public Health: the annual report of the Chief Medical Officer of the Department of Health for the year 1989*. London: HMSO, 1990; 119.

2 Nabarro JDN. Diabetes in the United Kingdom: some facts and figures. *Diabetic Med* 1987; **5**: 816-22.

3 Neil HAW, Mather HM, Thompson QV et al. The Oxford Community Diabetes Study: evidence for the increase in the prevalence of known diabetes in Great Britain. *Diabetic Med* 1987; **4**: 539-43.

4 Simmons D, Williams DRR, Powell MJ. Prevalence of diabetes in a predominantly Asian community: preliminary findings of the Coventry diabetes study. *Br Med J* 1989; **298**: 18-21.

5 Cruickshank JK. *Diabetes: contrasts between peoples of black (West African), Indian and white European origin*. In: Cruickshank JK, Beavers DG, editors. Ethnic Factors in Health and Disease. London: Wright, 1990; 289-304.

6 Keen H, Jarrett RJ, McCartney P. The ten year follow up of the Bedford survey (1962-1972): glucose tolerance and diabetes. *Diabetologia* 1982; **22**: 73-8.

7 Forrest RD, Jackson CA, Yudkin JS. Glucose intolerance and hypertension in North London: the Islington Diabetes Survey. *Diabetic Med* 1986; **3**: 338-42.

8   British Diabetic Association. *Diabetes in the United Kingdom*. London: BDA, 1988.

9   Houston A. *Retinopathy in the Poole area: an epidemiological inquiry*. In: Eschwege E, editor. Advances in diabetes epidemiology. INSERM Symposium No 22; 1982 May 3-7; Abbaye de Fontevraud (France). Amsterdam (Netherlands): Biomedical Press BV, 1982.

(b) Effectiveness of care

When purchasers of health care have assessed incidence and prevalence, they will need to be aware of what services might benefit diabetic patients, and of their potential effectiveness. Information about effectiveness is usually derived from research and evaluation of specific interventions. To assist purchasers, DH is supporting the publication of a series of bulletins summarising the known evidence on the effectiveness (including cost-effectiveness) and appropriate use of a wide range of medical care. They will be published between September 1991 and September 1993. In addition, DH's Directorate of Research and Development will support research intended to fill the gaps in knowledge about effectiveness. Guidelines on the most effective and appropriate treatment for people with diabetes have been developed in many hospitals and general practices. The Royal College of General Practitioners (RCGP) has produced a diabetes information folder[1], and the Department of General Practice at Exeter University has produced the Exeter diabetic protocol[2].

Apart from being aware of effectiveness, purchasers of health care will wish to be aware of the costs of different interventions in order to obtain the maximum benefit within the resources available. Economic appraisal provides an important tool in the decision making process for purchasers. For diabetes, one of the key purchasing issues is whether care should be based in general practice or in hospital. Unfortunately, the results of evaluations are inconclusive; some favour hospital-based care, others favour general practice[3]. The one evaluation that measured costs suggested that general practice care costs about half as much as hospital care. A second fundamental issue is the degree to which programmes to identify individuals with undiagnosed diabetes should be devised. The ratio between diagnosed and undiagnosed diabetes (almost exclusively non-insulin-dependent diabetes) in Districts has been put at between 1:1 and 1:2 by Williams and Tallis[4]. They went on to suggest that assessment of the benefits of early detection of diabetes requires considerable further clarification. Both the costs and the benefits of identifying, and perhaps treating, previously undiagnosed people with diabetes must be considered.

Quality of service and audit

Purchasers will match the need for care with available resources, set priorities, and then negotiate contracts for the provision of care. These will specify the quality of service expected from the provider. Clinical audit is one method of assessing the quality of service compared with the specified standards. The Royal College of Physicians (RCP), which is being funded by DH to undertake audit projects, is developing, together with the British Diabetic Association, a core data set for diabetes. Initially it will allow assessment of the quality of care given by one hospital, but later it will enable comparisons between hospitals. Clinicians will thus be able to decide whether they are providing the best possible care for their diabetic patients, and, where necessary, to improve their clinical practice and the organisation of the service. Districts will also need to ensure that the services they purchase are acceptable to patients.

References

1   Royal College of General Practitioners. *Diabetes Information Folder*. London: RCGP, 1988.
2   University of Exeter: Department of General Practice. *Exeter Diabetic Protocol: a handbook for general practitioners, practice nurses and practice staff*. Exeter: University of Exeter: Department of General Practice, 1985.
3   Wood J. A review of diabetic care initiatives in primary care settings. *Health Trends* 1990; **22**: 39–43.
4   Williams R, Tallis D. *Epidemiologically based needs assessment: report 1: diabetes mellitus*. National Health Service Management Executive, 1990. (DHA Project: Research Programme; Report 1).

(c) Outcomes of health care

In formulating a package of care, purchasers of health care will build up an expectation of the benefit to be derived, taking into account a patient's maintenance of, or improvement in, health, well-being, reassurance, satisfaction etc. The benefit is a cumulative effect of a variety of care in a variety of settings, eg at home by general practitioners and district nurses, and in hospital both as an inpatient and as an outpatient. It may manifest itself in the short term or after many years. Assessment of the outcome of health care involves assessment of the extent to which such benefit is achieved, and attributing the benefit to the care received.

The assessment is complex. To avoid each health authority having to develop its own methods of assessment, DH has commissioned a United Kingdom (UK) Clearing House on outcomes. It will collect, collate and disseminate the most up-to-date information on assessment of health care outcomes, and will be available to provide expert advice on resource requirements, methods of assessment, data collection systems, and analysis and interpretation of outcome studies.

Outcome measurement depends on accurate and appropriate information, not all of which is yet available. As far as diabetes is concerned, it also requires a population-based register of people with diabetes, and it may take some time for Districts to develop such registers. The complexities of measurement can be illustrated by describing the health outcomes expected from interventions for people with diabetes (see Table 4.2).

Preventing diabetes

The most effective interventions for the prevention of non-insulin-dependent diabetes are promotion of a balanced diet and advice to maintain a healthy weight, both targeted on the whole population. Effectiveness is demonstrated by a declining incidence of this form of diabetes. There are no known effective interventions which will reduce the incidence of insulin-dependent diabetes. However, stopping smoking will reduce the incidence of the complications of diabetes, particularly ischaemic heart disease and peripheral vascular disease. Assessment of the outcome of preventive services would require surveys to provide baseline information on people without diabetes, and on what proportion go on to develop it.

Identifying and managing people with diabetes

One outcome of health care is a reduction in the occurrence of, and hence admission to hospital for, ketoacidosis; another is blindness due to diabetes.

Table 4.2: *Service activity and desired health outcomes for people with diabetes mellitus*

Level at which intervention is made	Service activity	Desired health outcomes
Preventing diabetes	Education of people in general to adopt a healthy lifestyle and maintain a healthy weight	Decline in the incidence and prevalence of the sub-categories of diabetes in the population
Identifying those with diabetes	Case finding, registers	Increased proportion of people with diabetes diagnosed before the onset of complications
Management of the disease to prevent the development of complications, and to reduce the impairment and disability that result from it	Education of people with diabetes and their families Monitoring of the disease process—by agreed care plans Treatment interventions by: Primary care professionals Specialist diabetic teams Physicians Paediatricians Obstetricians Geriatricians Surgeons	Decreased incidence of short-term complications eg hypo- and hyperglycaemia Decreased proportion of people with diabetes admitted to hospital as a result of ketoacidosis Decreased intra-natal mortality rate for mothers with diabetes Decreased incidence of congenital malformation in children born to mothers with diabetes Declining incidence of: Ischaemic heart disease Peripheral vascular disease Cerebrovascular disease Diabetic eye disease Diabetic renal disease Diabetic neuropathy Reduction in preventable death Improved quality of life Reduction in handicap

Neither can be measured unless accurate data are provided respectively by the hospital (coding for cause of admission) and the local authority Social Services Department (registers of the blind). Any inaccuracy of the latter could be overcome by surveying samples of people with diabetes to determine what proportion becomes blind or visually impaired. A measure of outcome that may be more readily available is change in the incidence of diabetes-induced end-stage renal failure. At District level the numbers involved would be too small, but the incidence could be monitored at Regional level. The most effective way of reviewing some outcomes (eg diabetes of pregnancy and amputations) may be peer group review, using the confidential enquiry techniques that have been developed by the Royal Colleges. A review might examine the timing, appropriateness and effectiveness of interventions, and enable any lessons learned to be used to modify existing practice.

Until accurate and appropriate data for outcome measurement are available, the results of selected service activities, chosen because they have been shown to produce improvements in health, may have to be used to monitor purchasing decisions and the performance of contracts. For diabetes, the following service activities, or data derived from them, are likely to be associated with improved health, and could therefore serve as proxy measures for health care outcomes:

- The prevalence of diagnosed diabetes, compared with the expected prevalence for a population.

- The proportion of diagnosed diabetics with a locally agreed care plan.

- The proportion of practices within an FHSA providing diabetic clinics within a locally agreed protocol.

- The proportion of professional primary health care staff who have received postgraduate education about diabetes.

- The proportion of people with diabetes screened for the long-term complications of the disease.

- The proportion of people with diabetes admitted to hospital for diabetes-related episodes.

Conclusion

The NHS reforms require health authorities to purchase for their residents the highest quality service possible within the resources allocated to them. In order to do so they will need to assess the health care needs of their populations, be aware of the effectiveness of different types of care, and be able to measure the outcome of the care provided. As far as diabetes mellitus is concerned, considerable progress has been made in assessing needs for health care, in identifying the interventions likely to be effective, and in providing guidance on their appropriate use. However, the outcomes of such care cannot yet be measured accurately, but only implied. Only when they can be measured will it be possible to monitor the impact of purchasing decisions. Similar work needs to be undertaken for each aspect of health care.

(d) Outcomes of mental health care

DH's Mental Health Division recognised that a system of outcome indicators for mental health care is needed urgently to ensure that clinicians, DHAs and Directors of Public Health (DsPH) can monitor and evaluate mental health care. It therefore published, in October 1990, a review of the different classes of outcome indicators available[1]. This proposed a scheme of indicators for the broad diagnostic categories of schizophrenia, affective psychosis, neurosis, dementia, child psychiatry, forensic psychiatry, mental handicap, and alcohol and drug misuse. The factors on which they are based include whether incidence can be reduced, whether relapse rates and readmission rates can be reduced, whether total disability can be reduced, and whether there is avoidable mortality. The scheme is intended to form a basis for development by clinicians, researchers and planners for their own requirements, and not to be definitive or exhaustive.

Together with the Faculty of Public Health Medicine and the Royal College of Psychiatrists, the Division also organised two workshops to help DsPH and psychiatrists consider how to tackle the mental health component of the DPH's Annual Report as far as defining needs and measuring outcomes are concerned. The examination by Dr Stephen Farrow of the first 133 Annual Reports in 1989 revealed that only seven mentioned mental health. There are now encouraging signs that these ideas are being explored at local level by DsPH and psychiatrists, and DH is hoping to fund evaluative studies.

Reference

1   Jenkins R. Towards a system of total outcome indicators for mental health care. *Br J Psychiatry* 1990; **157**: 500-14.

5. COMMUNICABLE DISEASES

(a) AIDS and HIV infection

Monitoring and surveillance

The voluntary confidential reporting system in England and Wales continues to be operated by the Communicable Disease Surveillance Centre (CDSC) at Colindale. All available evidence suggests that the great majority of AIDS cases and known HIV-positive people are reported. Nonetheless CDSC staff constantly monitor other data sources to ensure that any under-reporting is identified and, as far as possible, eliminated.

However, many factors can affect an individual's decision whether to present for named HIV testing, so that laboratory reports of HIV infections give an incomplete, and possibly biased, picture of the development of the epidemic. The completeness of data from named testing may increase following publication of evidence[1] that there may now be clinical advantage in a seropositive person receiving early treatment to delay the onset of AIDS.

Against the background of improved treatment for HIV infection and opportunistic infections, the Chief Medical Officer issued a Press Notice to coincide with World AIDS Day (1 December) to encourage people who believed they had been exposed to risk of HIV infection to consider being tested for HIV antibody. The immediate result was an increase in the number of people requesting HIV antibody testing at the main clinics. The size of the response will be monitored during 1991.

The anonymous serosurvey programme

Data from named testing are now being complemented by the anonymous serosurvey programme which began in January 1990. The programme, funded by the Department of Health (DH) via the Medical Research Council (MRC), is concentrating initially on seroprevalence in pregnant women (using sera taken for rubella testing, and blood taken for Guthrie tests), attenders at genito-urinary medicine (GUM) clinics, and injecting drug users. DH mounted an extensive public information campaign, including literature in a number of ethnic minority languages, to ensure that the public was aware of the programme and knew that anyone wishing to opt out could do so. In the event the spontaneous objection rate has been extremely low. In addition, it is planned to begin a study of seroprevalance in some patients in general hospitals in 1991, during which the first results of the anonymous serosurvey programme are expected.

The shape of the epidemic

AIDS cases in England

Figure 5.1 shows that the flattening of the curve for reports of AIDS cases, seen in 1988 and 1989, was not maintained in 1990; the curve was steeper, although there were fluctuations between quarters. A possible explanation for the flattening and subsequent steepening of the curve is that earlier treatment with zidovudine postponed the development of AIDS in a substantial proportion of

Figure 5.1: *AIDS in the United Kingdom: cases by quarter of report and diagnosis, 1983-90*

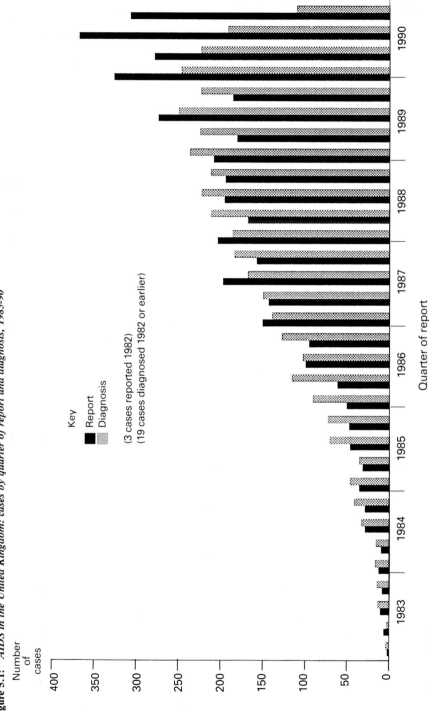

Source: CDSC

people. Some of these people have now developed AIDS, causing an increase in the number of reported cases.

Table 5.1 shows AIDS cases, and known deaths, in England to the end of 1990. The format of the table is different from that used in previous Reports. It includes time-banded data for the last two twelve-month periods so that the rate of growth for the different categories is easier to identify. Table 5.2 shows the distribution of reports of AIDS cases by Region. The marked concentration in the Thames Regions persists.

Heterosexuals with AIDS

The epidemic is in a complex phase. The number of cases in heterosexual people is increasing rapidly. Whether they themselves were infected during heterosexual intercourse or by using contaminated equipment when injecting drugs, they can transmit the virus to their heterosexual partners, and women can transmit the infection before or during birth to their babies. The heterosexual group is growing proportionally very quickly. It expanded by 115% in 1990, compared with an increase of 46% in AIDS cases in men who have sex with men. However, men who have sex with men still account for 81% of the cumulative total of AIDS cases.

Women with AIDS

The increasing importance of heterosexuals is emphasised by the more rapid growth in the number of cases in women than in men. Although men comprise 95% of cases, the proportional growth in the number of cases in women during 1990 was 119%, compared with 51% in men.

Survival with AIDS

The median survival time of people with AIDS is lengthening, from 10 months for cases diagnosed in 1984-86 to 20 months for cases diagnosed in 1987[2]. Most of this improved outlook is due to reduced mortality from pneumocystis pneumonia (PCP). Contributory factors probably include earlier presentation or earlier diagnosis, as well as zidovudine treatment and chemoprophylaxis with pentamidine and co-trimoxazole to prevent PCP.

International situation

Comparisons between countries are difficult because of differences in the completeness of the reporting systems. The global dominance by the USA persists, with 154,791 reports to WHO by the end of 1990. Comparable figures for Africa were 80,583, and for Europe 42,113. Table 5.3 shows the ranking of the 12 European Community (EC) countries by cumulative totals of AIDS cases per million population. The United Kingdom (UK) was ranked ninth in 1990, as it was in 1989.

HIV-seropositive people

Table 5.4 shows reported seropositive people, in the same new format as Table 5.1. Most of these seropositive people are also included in the tables of AIDS

Table 5.1: *AIDS cases and known deaths by exposure category and date of report, England, to 31 December 1990*
(Numbers subject to revision as further data are received or duplicates identified)

How persons probably acquired the virus	Jan 89-Dec 89		Jan 90-Dec 90		Jan 82-Dec 90		
	Cases	Deaths	Cases	Deaths	Cases	Deaths	
	Number	Number	Number	Number	Number	Number	%
Sexual intercourse:							
between men	617	240	901	222	3086	1702	55
between men and women							
'high risk' partner*	7	5	9	2	28	17	61
other partner abroad**	49	31	92	23	187	82	44
other partner UK	6	2	12	1	22	6	27
Injecting drug use (IDU)	17	9	57	18	101	48	47
IDU & sexual intercourse between men	9	3	20	6	60	31	52
Blood							
Blood factor (eg haemophiliacs)	39	20	54	22	205	138	67
Blood or tissue transfer (eg transfusion)							
Abroad	5	5	12	3	36	22	61
UK	7	5	7	4	25	19	76
Mother to child	2	1	13	1	32	12	37
Other/undetermined	12	5	12	8	35	23	66
Total	770	326	1189	310	3817	2100	55

* Includes men and women who had sex with injecting drug users, or with those infected by contaminated blood, and women who had sex with bisexual men.

** Includes persons without other identified risks who are from, or who have lived in, countries where the major route of HIV-1 transmission is through sexual intercourse between men and women.

Source: CDSC

Table 5.2: *AIDS cases and known deaths reported by Region of reporter, England, to 31 December 1990*
(Numbers subject to revision as further data are received or duplicates identified)

Region	Jan 89-Dec 89				Jan 90-Dec 90				Jan 82-Dec 90			
	Cases		Deaths		Cases		Deaths		Cases		Deaths	
	Number	%	Number	%	Number	%	Number	%	Number	%	Number	%
Northern	9	1	3	1	28	2	5	2	83	2	46	2
Yorkshire	27	3	13	4	39	3	16	5	112	3	67	3
Trent	15	2	4	1	24	2	7	2	80	2	43	2
E Anglia	11	1	9	3	7	1	1	1	42	1	30	1
NW Thames	331	43	119	37	500	42	84	27	1621	42	797	38
NE Thames	144	19	49	15	223	19	64	21	733	19	395	19
SE Thames	96	13	57	18	150	13	43	14	453	12	275	13
SW Thames	33	4	21	6	43	4	21	7	141	4	100	5
Wessex	16	2	7	2	31	3	16	5	94	2	62	3
Oxford	13	2	8	2	28	2	7	2	83	2	48	2
S Western	17	2	8	2	19	2	10	3	76	2	51	2
W Midlands	23	3	10	3	33	3	13	4	91	2	54	3
Mersey	6	1	5	2	16	1	7	2	52	1	37	2
N Western	29	4	13	4	48	4	16	5	156	4	95	5
Total	770	100*	326	100*	1189	100*	310	100*	3817	100*	2100	100*

* Total may not add up to 100 because of rounding.

Source: CDSC

Table 5.3: *AIDS cases reported to WHO by EC countries: cumulative totals at 31 December 1990* (USA figures shown for comparison)

Country	Number of cases	Population (millions)	Cumulative cases per million population
Spain	7047	39	181
France	9718	55	177
Denmark	705	5	141
Italy	7576	58	131
Netherlands	1487	15	99
Germany*	5500	60	92
Belgium	764	10	76
Luxembourg	30	<1	75
UK	3884	57	68
Portugal	522	11	47
Ireland	161	4	40
Greece	375	10	37
USA	154791	230	673

* Although Germany is now integrated only figures for the former West Germany are available.

Table 5.4: *HIV antibody positive people by exposure category and date of report, England, to 31 December 1990*
(Numbers subject to revision as further data are received or duplicates identified)

How persons probably acquired the virus	Jan 89-Dec 89			Jan 90-Dec 90			Jan 82-Dec 90				
	Male	Female	NK†	Male	Female	NK†	Male	Female	NK†	Total	%
Sexual intercourse:											
between men	1195	—	—	1433	—	—	8130	—	—	8130	63
between men and women											
'high risk' partner*	5	25	—	6	27	—	20	130	—	150	1
other partner abroad**	66	52	1	112	99	1	324	242	7	573	4
other partner UK	5	4	—	9	18	—	30	36	2	68	<1
under investigation	35	24	—	43	43	—	124	113	—	237	2
Injecting drug use (IDU)	126	40	—	132	45	1	725	331	5	1061	8
IDU & sexual intercourse between men	18	—	—	18	—	—	152	—	—	152	1
Blood											
Blood factor (eg haemophiliacs)	25	2	—	34	—	—	1095	6	1	1102	8
Blood or tissue transfer (eg transfusion)											
Abroad/UK	11	7	1	7	11	—	63	58	2	123	1
Mother to child	10	5	—	19	15	1	54	35	3	92	1
Other/undetermined	159	44	4	102	23	7	1071	148	78	1297	10
Total	1655	203	6	1915	281	10	11788	1099	98	12985	100

† NK = Not known.

* Includes men and women who had sex with injecting drug users, or with those infected by contaminated blood, and women who had sex with bisexual men.

** Includes persons without other identified risks who are from, or who have lived in, countries where the major route of HIV-1 transmission is through sexual intercourse between men and women.

Source: CDSC

Table 5.5: *HIV antibody positive people reported by Region of reporter, England, to 31 December 1990*
(Numbers subject to revision as further data are received or duplicates identified)

Region	Jan 89-Dec 89		Jan 90-Dec 90		Jan 82-Dec 90	
	Number	%	Number	%	Number	%
Northern	32	2	46	2	357	3
Yorkshire	40	2	59	3	395	3
Trent	51	3	103	5	394	3
E Anglia	29	1	23	1	203	2
NW Thames	658	35	905	41	4682	36
NE Thames	462	25	371	17	2507	19
SE Thames	243	13	240	11	1640	13
SW Thames	77	4	103	5	425	3
Wessex	41	2	47	2	318	2
Oxford	37	2	36	2	389	3
S Western	44	3	56	3	310	2
W Midlands	46	3	106	5	495	4
Mersey	20	1	19	1	190	1
N Western	84	4	92	4	680	5
Total	1864	100*	2206	100*	12985	100*

* Total may not add up to 100 because of rounding.

Source: CDSC

116

cases. Even allowing for this overlap, for the fact that some of these seropositive people have died, and for some undetectable duplicates, it is virtually certain that the true total of seropositive people is substantially higher than that shown, as asymptomatic people may not present themselves for testing. The Regional distribution of seropositive people is shown in Table 5.5. As with AIDS cases, the marked concentration in the Thames Regions persists.

HIV-seropositive heterosexuals

As with AIDS cases, there is evidence of rapid growth of the number of people heterosexually infected. Reports in this group increased by 65% during 1990, compared with 20% for men who have sex with men. While the overall preponderance of reports of the latter group persists, it is less marked than for cases of AIDS. This evidence supports DH's earlier statements that HIV infection would spread into the general heterosexually active population from the other risk behaviour groups unless people adopted safer sexual and injecting drug use practices.

HIV/AIDS in injecting drug misusers

There was a 235% increase in the number of AIDS cases reported amongst injecting drug misusers in 1990 (57) compared with 1989 (17). 56% of the cumulative total of 101 cases were reported in 1990. However, there was no appreciable rate of increase in the reported numbers of HIV-positive individuals in this risk group during the year. Of the cumulative total of 1,061 reports, 17% were made in 1990, a similar proportion to that in 1989. Studies to be published in 1991 may help to assess the rate of growth of seropositivity in this population. Other issues concerning HIV infection and drug misuse are described in Chapter 2.

HIV/AIDS probably contracted through heterosexual intercourse abroad

Table 5.1 shows that the number of reported AIDS cases due to heterosexual transmission abroad increased by almost 90% in 1990 compared with 1989. Combined reports for the years 1989 and 1990 account for 75% of the cumulative total of known cases transmitted in this manner. Table 5.4 shows that the number of HIV-positive reports in this transmission group also increased rapidly, by about 80% in 1990 compared with 1989. The total number of HIV-positive heterosexuals in this category is 573, of whom 37% were reported in 1990. These reports include people without any other identified risks who are from, or who have lived in, countries where the major route of HIV-1 transmission is heterosexual intercourse between men and women. The rapid growth in numbers in both sexes in these categories underlines the importance of increasing the awareness of the risks of HIV infection in people travelling abroad, and of encouraging these people to take appropriate measures to protect themselves from infection.

HIV/AIDS cases in recipients of blood and blood products

The cumulative number of AIDS cases in haemophiliacs was 205 by the end of 1990, 67% of whom had died. Approximately a quarter of these were reported in 1990, a slight increase on the 1989 figure. The total number of known HIV-positive haemophiliacs (which includes the 205 known AIDS cases) was 1,102 by the end of 1990. Although some of the HIV-positive haemophiliacs and blood transfusion recipients shown in Table 5.4 were reported in 1989 and 1990, the vast majority were infected before the introduction of HIV testing of blood donations and heat treatment of blood products in 1985.

The safety of the blood supply and appropriate sterilisation of surgical instruments are not assured in all countries. A significant number of HIV-positive people and AIDS cases were infected by blood transfusions abroad, and people travelling abroad need to be aware of these risks.

HIV in blood donations

During 1990 screening of blood donations with the anti-HIV-1 + 2 combined test commenced in the UK. Of the 2.82 million donations tested, 1.73 million were tested by this method (61%). 33 donations, 12 of which were from women, were found to be HIV-1-seropositive (0.0012%)—see Table 5.6. Among new donors, 18 (five women) were HIV-1-seropositive in 352,704 donations (0.005%), and one individual was HIV-2-seropositive.

Table 5.6 also shows comparable figures since HIV-1 testing was introduced in the Blood Transfusion Service in the autumn of 1985, including details of risk category. It is hoped that information on the eight donors for whom it has not been possible to define risk activities may become available during 1991 when they attend for interview.

Table 5.6: *HIV in blood donations in the United Kingdom, 1985-90*

Risk activity	1985 M	1985 F	1986 M	1986 F	1987 M	1987 F	1988 M	1988 F	1989 M	1989 F	1990 M	1990 F
Homosexual/bisexual	8		23		11		11		11		10	
Intravenous drug user	5		9	1			1		3	1		
Sexual partner at risk			4	6		5	4	2	2	6	3	4
Blood transfusion				1					?1			
Sexual relations abroad	1		2		2				2		1*	2
Denies risk/presumed heterosexual transmission			2	1	2		1	2	4	2	2	1
No information or not traced			2		2		1	1	1	2	5	3
Others: Multiple sexual partners			1		1					1	1	2
Tattoo			1		1							
Total	14		44	9	19	5	18	5	24	12	22	12

* HIV-2-seropositive.

Source: National Blood Transfusion Service Directorate

HIV infection in health care settings

During 1990 health care professionals expressed concern about possible transmission of HIV from patients to staff in health care settings, despite evidence that the risk of such transmission was very low. Their attention was drawn to the *Guidance for Clinical Health Care Workers*[3] and revised guidelines on HIV from the Advisory Committee on Dangerous Pathogens[4], both published in January 1990. A sub-group of the Chief Medical Officer's Expert Advisory Group on AIDS began to review its 1988 guidance on the working practices of HIV-infected health care workers[5]. A possible case of transmission of HIV from a dentist with AIDS to a patient during an operative procedure was reported from the USA. Revised guidance on HIV antibody testing of donors of tissues and organs for transplantation was issued in April[6].

Public education

Public education about HIV and AIDS continued at national and local levels as part of the Government's commitment to preventing the transmission of HIV infection.

National initiatives

The Health Education Authority (HEA) developed further television and press campaigns to inform the public about the risks of infection, and in February 1990 launched a campaign featuring well known experts in HIV and AIDS, including the Chief Medical Officer. The campaign built on the conclusions of the expert symposium held in November 1989, and provided information about the ways HIV infection could be transmitted and the steps people could take to protect themselves and others.

The campaign aimed at homosexual men continued throughout 1990, and was expanded to include advertising in a range of magazines, supported by leaflets and promotional materials, aimed at persuading homosexual men to sustain safer sexual behaviour. Bisexual men were a key audience, and in February 1990 a campaign directed towards them was launched in a number of male orientated publications. Advertising highlighted the risks from unprotected anal inter-course, and was supported by a telephone helpline run in conjunction with the National AIDS Helpline.

The HEA developed a further summer radio and press campaign to remind holiday travellers of the risk of infection, and encourage them to use condoms if they had penetrative sex with new partners, either at home or abroad. The latest phase of the mass media campaign was launched in December 1990 and built on the success of the 'Experts' campaign. Personal testimonies from a range of individuals infected with HIV were used to persuade people to acknowledge the risks and to review their own sexual behaviour. A cinema campaign reminding young people about condom use was launched simultaneously. The National AIDS Helpline, which supports the campaigns and provides confidential advice to those worried about HIV and AIDS, received a record number of calls, dealing with 750,000 enquiries from the public in 1990.

Local initiatives

During 1989/90 the Government provided funding to Regional and District Health Authorities (RHAs and DHAs) for the development of local HIV prevention work to complement the national campaign and to focus on local needs. Each District was asked to appoint an HIV prevention co-ordinator to ensure effective planning and co-ordination of the prevention work in the statutory and voluntary sectors. A highly successful national seminar for these co-ordinators was held on 19 and 20 November 1990. This helped to place their work in a national context and encouraged the exchange of ideas and experience. Local campaigns by health authorities, focusing on the prevention of drug abuse, including the risks of HIV infection, were also financed by the Government. Other Government Departments continued to develop HIV and AIDS educational work within their own spheres of interest.

Finance for HIV/AIDS treatment, care and prevention services

In the year beginning April 1990, DH allocated £129.5 million from the Hospital and Community Health Service budget to support HIV and AIDS treatment, care and prevention services. In 1991/92 the allocation will be increased to £137.3 million. RHAs distributed the money to their Districts to use in accordance with the following Ministerial priorities:

- Development of local community-based HIV prevention initiatives.

- Development of drug misuse and genito-urinary medicine services to enable them to cope with the additional pressures presented by HIV.

- Hospital treatment and community care of people with HIV disease.

- Improvement of local monitoring and surveillance of progression of the disease.

- Improvement of protection of donated blood, organs and tissues, and infection control.

Progress in implementation is monitored through the Department's routine accountability and review processes. The AIDS (Control) Act 1987[7], which was annexed to 1990 planning statements, requires RHAs and DHAs to publish annual reports on:

i.   Provision of local HIV and AIDS services.

ii. How money allocated for these services has been spent.

The Regional reports are sent to the Department in July.

During the year the Department also allocated money for HIV/AIDS projects, from the same budget, to the Special Health Authorities, the Public Health Laboratory Service (PHLS), the English National Board and local authorities. This last allocation was for initiatives jointly financed with health authorities.

Service provision

The AIDS (Control) Act 1987[7] reports show an encouraging development of innovative inpatient, outpatient and community-based services, often provided in collaboration with voluntary agencies or local authorities. The increase in collaborative working has been facilitated by the appointment of Regional and District HIV prevention co-ordinators. It is encouraging that progress is being made in looking at ways in which services can attract particular groups, such as women with children and drug users. During 1991 additional pressures on the services may include more people coming forward for testing in order to take advantage of the possible benefits of early intervention.

References

1 Volberding P. HIV infection as a disease: The medical indications for early diagnosis. *Journal of Acquired Immune Deficiency Syndromes* 1989; **2**: 421-5.

2 Peters BS et al. Changing disease patterns in patients with AIDS in a referral centre in the United Kingdom: the changing face of AIDS. *Br Med J* 1991; **302**: 203-7.

3 Expert Advisory Group on AIDS. *Guidance for clinical health care workers: protection against infection with HIV and hepatitis viruses.* London: HMSO, 1990.

4 Advisory Committee on Dangerous Pathogens. *HIV: the causative agent of AIDS and related conditions: second revision of guidelines.* Department of Health, 1990.

5 Expert Advisory Group on AIDS. *AIDS: HIV-infected health care workers: report of the recommendations of the Expert Advisory Group on AIDS.* London: HMSO, 1988. Chairman: Sir Donald Acheson.

6 Department of Health. *HIV infection, tissue banks and organ donation.* London: Department of Health 1990. (Professional Letter: PL/CMO(90)2).

7 *AIDS (Control) Act 1987.* London: HMSO, 1987.

(b) Other sexually transmitted diseases

Implementation of the recommendations of the Working Group set up under the chairmanship of Mr Alan Monks in 1988 continued in 1990[1]. Several Regions conducted their own surveys into GUM services and a number of clinics were refurbished or moved to new premises. New clinics were opened in some Districts.

The General Assembly of the International Union of Venereal Diseases and Treponematoses was held in London in May.

Statistical returns

By the beginning of 1989, all clinics were making returns on Form KC60, which was brought into use in either the second or third quarter of 1988. Some of the returns for 1988 were made on the old Form SBH60, which had fewer categories than Form KC60, and the equivalent Form KC60 categories were estimated. For some categories the approximations involved in this estimation make comparisons between 1988 and 1989 difficult. Where this is the case, data from the last two quarters of each year have been used to examine the underlying trends. Some clinics are still not reporting the number of homosexually acquired infections, and the figures quoted below should be regarded as estimates. The KC60 returns for the whole of 1989 are listed in Table 5.7, and Figure 5.2 shows the breakdown of new cases seen during the year. The total number of new cases seen in 1989 was 572,943, a 2% increase compared with 1988.

Figure 5.2 *New cases seen at NHS genito-urinary medicine clinics, England, 1989—breakdown by condition*

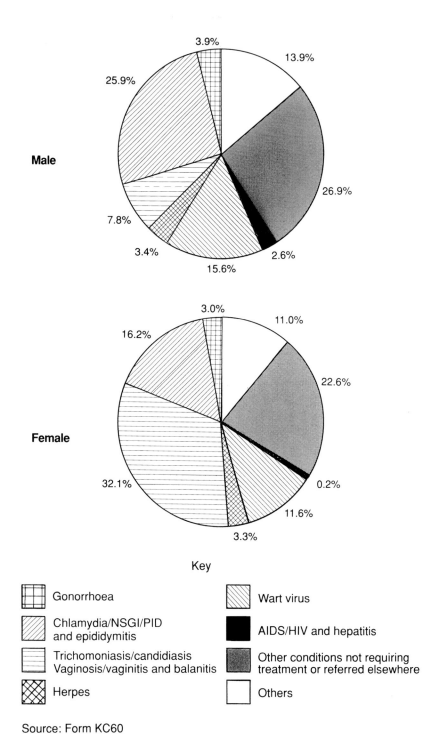

Key

Gonorrhoea

Wart virus

Chlamydia/NSGI/PID and epididymitis

AIDS/HIV and hepatitis

Trichomoniasis/candidiasis Vaginosis/vaginitis and balanitis

Other conditions not requiring treatment or referred elsewhere

Herpes

Others

Source: Form KC60

Table 5.7: *Sexually transmitted diseases reported by NHS genito-urinary medicine clinics in England in the year ending 31 December 1989*

Condition	Males		Females	
All syphilis	923		488	
Infectious syphilis		269		122
All gonorrhoea	11346		8415	
Post-pubertal uncomplicated		10708		6986
Chancroid/Donovanosis/LGV	67		21	
Other chlamydia (excluding PID and chlamydial infections with arthritis)	16081		20880	
Post-pubertal uncomplicated		12752		17515
Pelvic infection and epididymitis	1326		4954	
Non-specific urethritis and related diseases	57894		19366	
Chlamydial infections/NSU with arthritis	456		44	
Trichomoniasis	316		7437	
Vaginosis/vaginitis/balanitis	8539		30865	
Candidiasis	9811		48382	
Scabies/pediculosis	5344		2142	
Herpes—all	9906		9382	
Herpes simplex—first attack		5792		6611
Herpes simplex—recurrence		4114		2771
Wart virus infections—all	45804		32342	
Wart virus infection—first attack		27448		23506
Wart virus infection—recurrence		18356		8836
Viral hepatitis	548		59	
HIV/AIDS	7130		470	
Other conditions requiring treatment*	38861		31466	
Other episodes not requiring treatment	74179		56797	
Other conditions referred elsewhere	4549		6353	
Total new cases seen	293080		279863	

* Includes epidemiological treatment of trichomoniasis, vaginosis, vaginitis, balanitis and candidiasis.

Gonorrhoea

The trend in the incidence of gonorrhoea since 1977 is shown in Figure 5.3. Reports of male gonorrhoea fell from 36,908 cases in 1977 to 28,759 in 1985, followed by a much greater fall over the next three years to 10,847 cases in 1988. Female gonorrhoea decreased from 21,826 cases in 1977 to 16,255 in 1986, and then halved over the following two years to 7,891 cases in 1988. These trends were not maintained in 1989; a total of 19,761 cases were reported, compared with 18,738 in 1988. It is probably more reliable to compare the figures for post-pubertal uncomplicated gonorrhoea. These show an increase from 17,062 cases in 1988 to 17,694 cases in 1989. The increase in males (4%) was slightly greater than that in females (3%). About 6% of all infections in men were homosexually acquired. The total number of reports was less than that in 1987. This overall increase masks a variation within and between Regions. The Thames Regions, and particular clinics within those Regions, showed the most marked increase in reports of gonorrhoea, whilst other clinics and other Regions continued to show a decline.

Figure 5.3: *All gonorrhoea: number of new cases seen at NHS genito-urinary medicine clinics, England, 1977-89*

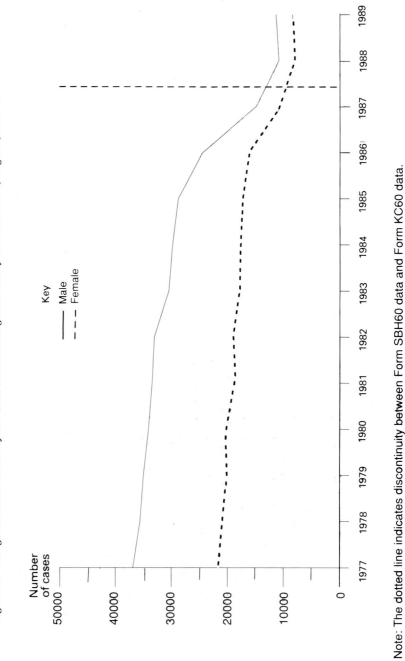

Note: The dotted line indicates discontinuity between Form SBH60 data and Form KC60 data.

Source: Forms SBH60 and KC60

Figure 5.4: *Infectious syphilis: number of new cases seen at NHS genito-urinary medicine clinics, England, 1977-89*

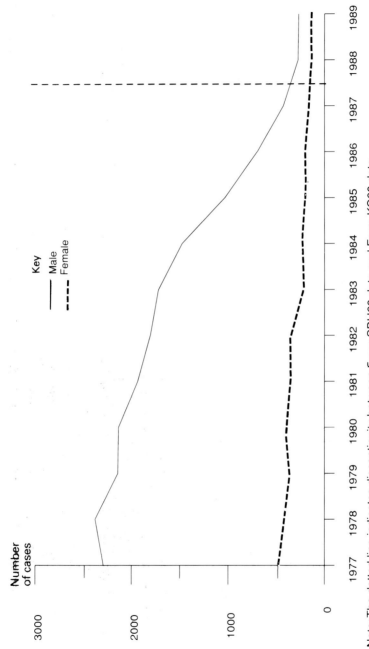

Note: The dotted line indicates discontinuity between Form SBH60 data and Form KC60 data.

Source: Forms SBH60 and KC60

Where it is considered wise to treat contacts of gonorrhoea without micro-biological confirmation of the diagnosis, the case is reported as 'epidemiological treatment of suspected gonorrhoea'. In 1989, this heading accounted for 9.5% of cases.

Syphilis

The trend in the incidence of infectious syphilis since 1977 is shown in Figure 5.4. Infectious syphilis in males decreased from 2,291 cases in 1977 to 429 in 1987, and to 275 in 1988. Reports of infectious syphilis in females also decreased, from 468 cases in 1977 to 160 in 1987, and to 117 in 1988. In 1989, the total number of cases of infectious syphilis remained stable in both males and females, but the total number of cases of all syphilis rose from 1,242 to 1,411. About 19% of all infections in men were homosexually acquired. Cases treated on epidemiological grounds (as defined in the previous paragraph) accounted for 5.2% of the total.

Chlamydia and non-specific genital infection

Until 1987, reports of chlamydial disease were included in the figure for non-specific genital infection. Form KC60 now includes separate headings for 'chlamydia', 'pelvic infection and epididymitis' and 'non-specific urethritis'. In 1989, the total number of reports under the heading 'chlamydia' was 36,961. The comparable figure for 1988 was 36,008. These figures include 100 reports of chlamydia ophthalmia neonatorum in 1988 and 42 in 1989. Homosexually acquired disease accounted for 1.4% of cases in men, and epidemiological treatment for 5,606 cases (15.2%).

In 1988, there were 75,668 cases of non-specific genital infection other than those attributable to chlamydia. In 1989, this had increased by 2.1% to 77,260. Comparison of the last two quarters of each year showed a slight decrease of 1%, and this may be a more reliable figure as all returns in these quarters were made on Form KC60.

In 1987, a total of 131,384 reports were made under the heading of non-specific genital infections. Comparable figures for 1988 and 1989 were 117,397 and 120,014 respectively. In 1989, chlamydia was identified or suspected in 48% of women and 22% of men in this category.

Pelvic inflammatory disease and epididymitis

In 1989 there were 4,954 cases of pelvic inflammatory disease (PID). On comparison of the data for the last two quarters of 1988 and 1989, this represents an increase of about 3%. 231 (4.7%) were reported as gonococcal alone, 602 (12.2%) as chlamydial, and 86 (1.7%) as mixed. No organism was found in 4,035 (81.4%). During 1989 there was a marked increase in the number of cases of gonococcal PID, rising from 88 in the first two quarters to 143 in the last two quarters.

A total of 1,326 cases of epididymitis was reported: 95 were gonococcal (7.2%), 196 chlamydial (14.8%), 33 were mixed (2.5%) and no organism was found in 1,002 (75.6%). Although chlamydia still accounted for a greater number of cases than gonorrhoea, there was a marked increase during the year in the number of cases of gonococcal epididymitis. 17 cases were reported in the first six months of the year and 78 in the final six months.

Trichomoniasis

Reports of trichomoniasis have been decreasing since the early 1980s, a decline mirroring that seen in the classical sexually transmitted diseases, gonorrhoea and syphilis. In the case of trichomoniasis, this decline continued in 1989, with a decrease of about 9.5% compared with 1988.

Genital warts and herpes

Viral conditions account for an increasing proportion of the diseases seen in GUM clinics; they place greater workload demands than the classical bacterial diseases because of the nature of the treatment, and because of their tendency to recur. Reports of genital warts and herpes have not shown the same recent decrease as other conditions. The possible slight decline in the total number of cases of herpes noted in 1988 was not confirmed in 1989. Comparison of the last two quarters of each year shows an increase of about 4% in cases of primary herpes, and a slightly larger increase (7.4%) in cases of recurrent herpes. There was also an increase in the number of patients with recurrent wart virus infection (9.3%), but the number with first attacks of wart virus decreased by about 6.7%. The ratio of recurrent to first attacks was 1:1.8 for herpes and 1:1.9 for wart virus.

Candidiasis, vaginosis/vaginitis and balanitis

This is a group of conditions in which infection is not necessarily sexually transmitted. There was a 7.1% increase in cases of candidiasis between 1988 and 1989. This may be due to more patients being referred to GUM clinics for treatment rather than a real increase. Vaginosis and balanitis were specified for the first time in Form KC60. If the last two quarters of each year are compared, there was an increase of 11.8% between 1988 and 1989.

HIV infection

CDSC runs a voluntary confidential reporting system for HIV infection and AIDS. The data are discussed on pages 109-118.

GUM clinics are an important source of confidential advice, counselling and antibody testing for patients suspected of having HIV infection and for the 'worried well', and this has a significant impact on their workload. Since the introduction of Form KC60, cases of HIV infection on first presentation, asymptomatic infection on subsequent presentations, and first presentations of symptomatic HIV disease and AIDS have been recorded. In 1989, the total number of cases recorded in these categories was 7,600. The number recorded in the final quarter of 1989 increased by about 38% compared with the number seen in the final quarter of 1988.

Other conditions

These groups accounted for 204,662 cases in 1989, 35.7% of all cases seen. A number of conditions which are now reported in their own right may previously have been described as 'other conditions requiring treatment'. Reporting practices may not have been uniform and there is a lack of certainty about the total under this heading in 1988. Comparison of the last two quarters of 1988 and 1989 suggest that the number of cases under this heading has increased by about 6%. 'Other conditions not requiring treatment' still constitutes the largest single category, representing 22.9% of all cases seen. In 1988, there was an increase in 'other conditions referred elsewhere', and this trend continued in 1989 with an increase of 30.4% in cases in this category.

Conclusion

The reassuring downward trend in sexually transmitted diseases in the mid-1980s, which was discussed in the Reports for 1988 and 1989, was not maintained in 1989. There was an increase in the total number of new cases seen.

The bulk of this increase is due to HIV infection and AIDS, to conditions that are not necessarily sexually transmitted, and to viral infections, particularly recurrences. However, for the first time in many years, there was an increase in gonorrhoea and a levelling out of reports of infectious syphilis. The recent decrease in chlamydia/non-specific genital infections did not continue, although trichomoniasis did continue to decline. Improved services might attract patients previously treated by general practitioners (GPs), but there is evidence that increased reporting of gonorrhoea and syphilis is confined to relatively few clinics in urban areas. A number of clinics have reported a particularly disturbing increase in disease that is homosexually acquired. Similar trends have been reported from parts of the USA[2] and from Europe[3], and it is suggested that groups who modified their behaviour as a result of the threat of HIV infection and AIDS may now be reverting to previous patterns of behaviour. This underlines the need for continuing publicity and education, not only about HIV infection and AIDS, but also about sexual health in general. In particular, new ways must be found to reinforce 'safer sex' messages.

References

1 Department of Health and Social Security. *Report of the Working Group to examine workloads in genito-urinary medicine clinics*. London: Department of Health and Social Security, 1988.
2 Handsfield HH, Schwebke J. Trends in sexually transmitted diseases in homosexually active men in King County, Washington, 1980-1990. *Sex Trans Dis* 1990; **17**: 211-5.
3 van den Hoek JAR, van Griensven GJP, Coutinho RA. Increase in unsafe homosexual behaviour [Letter]. *Lancet* 1990; **ii**: 179-80.

(c) Foodborne diseases

Committee on the Microbiological Safety of Food

The Committee on the Microbiological Safety of Food, under the chairmanship of Sir Mark Richmond FRS, was established in February 1989 by the Secretary of State for Health, the Minister for Agriculture, and the Secretaries of State for Scotland, Wales and Northern Ireland to advise on matters remitted to it by Ministers relating to the microbiological safety of food, and on such matters as it considers need investigation. Ministers asked the Committee to consider specific questions relating to the increasing incidence of microbiological illnesses of foodborne origin, particularly from salmonella, listeria and campylobacter; to establish whether this is linked to changes in agriculture and food production, food technology and distribution, retailing, catering, and food handling in the home; and to recommend action where appropriate.

Part I of the Committee's Report was published in February 1990[1], together with the Government's response[2]; Part II will be published early in January 1991. Part I included a review of the epidemiological data on salmonella, campylobacter and listeria, examined the arrangements in England and Wales for the epidemiological surveillance of humans and food animals, and for outbreak management. It made a detailed appraisal of microbiological hazards in relation to poultry meat production, food manufacturing processes and the activities of small food processing enterprises. The principal recommendations, which were addressed variously to the Government, enforcement agencies, professional bodies and the food industry, were:

i.   the establishment of a national system of food-related microbiological surveillance, and in particular a new permanent committee structure to oversee surveillance, interpret its results, and give Ministers independent advice on policy;

ii. that food processing should be designed on the principles of the Hazard Analysis and Critical Control Point (HACCP) system, which involves the identification of those points which are critical in relation to the microbiological contamination of food, and of where controls can most effectively be applied;

iii. that food hygiene training within all sectors of the food industry was essential in reducing the risk of food poisoning to the consumer;

iv. that there was a need to develop common standards of enforcement of food safety legislation throughout the country; and

v.   that there should be close control and oversight of certain more sensitive food processes and of certain types of food business, preferably involving licensing requirements relating to the risks involved.

Notifications of food poisoning

In 1990, notifications of food poisoning for England and Wales made to the Office of Population Censuses and Surveys (OPCS) came to the corrected figure of 52,145. This represents a very small decrease compared with the figure for 1989 (52,557)—see Figure 5.5 and Table 5.8. It is the first time since 1986 that the upward trend in notifications of food poisoning appears to have stopped.

Figure 5.5: *Notifications of food poisoning*, England and Wales, 1982-90*

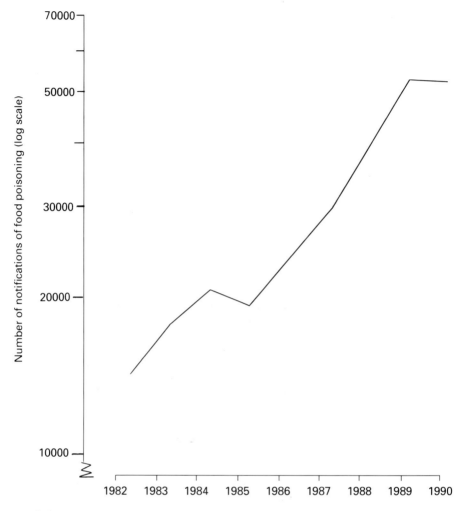

*Statutorily notified to OPCS and ascertained by other means.

Source: OPCS

Salmonellosis

The total number of reports of isolations of salmonella confirmed by the Division of Enteric Pathogens (DEP) at the Central Public Health Laboratory in 1990 was 30,112, compared with 29,998 in 1989. During 1990 there was a substantial decline in reports of isolations of *Salmonella typhimurium* and a smaller decline in reports of other serotypes, with the exception of *Salmonella enteritidis* (see Table 5.9). The marginal increase in the total number of serotypes reported includes a substantial increase for *Salmonella enteritidis PT4* of 25% compared with 1989. This organism causes over 50% of human salmonellosis.

Table 5.8: *Food poisoning: notifications in England and Wales, 1982-90*

Year	Total*
1982	14253
1983	17735
1984	20702
1985	19242
1986	23948
1987	29331
1988	39713
1989	52557
1990	52145

* Statutorily notified to OPCS and ascertained by other means.

Source: OPCS

In October 1990, DH issued a Press Release[3] stressing to caterers and consumers the importance of achieving high standards of food hygiene in catering establishments and in the home. The Department reminded everyone to avoid eating raw eggs or uncooked dishes made from them, and that vulnerable groups, such as the elderly, the sick, babies, toddlers and pregnant women, should consume only eggs that are thoroughly cooked until the white and yolk are solid. Attention was also drawn to the need to avoid raw poultry meat contaminating other foods in the kitchen, and to cook all poultry meat thoroughly.

Table 5.9: *Salmonella in humans, England and Wales, January to December (inclusive) 1989 and 1990*

Serotype	1989		1990	
	Confirmed reports	Acquired abroad (%)	Confirmed reports	Acquired abroad (%)
S. enteritidis all phage types	15773	2017 (13)	18840	1282 (7)
[Phage type 4	12931	1467 (11)	16151	946 (6)]
S. typhimurium	7306	619 (8)	5451	357 (7)
Other serotypes	6919	1930 (28)	5821	1669 (29)
All serotypes	29998	4566 (15)	30112	3308 (11)

Source: DEP Data

Campylobacter enteritis

Campylobacter continue to be the most commonly identified bacteria causing acute gastro-enteritis in humans. In 1990 there were 34,552 laboratory reports of campylobacter faecal isolations to CDSC, compared with 32,526 in 1989 (see Table 5.10). Most of these reports were of sporadic isolations. However, in 1990 there were a number of small outbreaks of illness associated with the contamination of bottled milk caused by magpies and jackdaws pecking the foil tops[4,5]. DH and the Ministry of Agriculture, Fisheries and Food (MAFF) discussed this problem with the Dairy Industry with a view to introducing measures in the spring of 1991 to prevent these scavenging birds contaminating the milk.

Table 5.10: *Laboratory reports of campylobacter faecal isolates to CDSC, England and Wales, 1980–90*

Year	Total reports
1980	8956
1981	12168
1982	12797
1983	17278
1984	21018
1985	23572
1986	24809
1987	27310
1988	28761
1989	32526
1990	34522*

* Provisional data.

Source: Communicable Disease Surveillance Centre, PHLS

Listeriosis

Since the number of reported cases of listeriosis in England and Wales reached a peak in 1988 (281 cases), there has been a continued and dramatic fall in the number of cases reported (see Figure 5.6). In the latter half of 1989, following DH's Press Release in July of that year[6] advising pregnant women and immunocompromised persons not to eat any type of pâté, the number of cases of listeriosis reported started to decrease, falling to 244 for the year. In 1990, the number of cases fell further to 116. This is very heartening and it is hoped that this downward trend will continue.

Conclusion

In 1990, the number of notifications of food poisoning decreased slightly compared with 1989. This encouraging trend is counterbalanced by the continued increase in reported isolations of *Salmonella enteritidis PT4*, the organism which causes most cases of human salmonellosis and which is associated with poultry meat and eggs. Although MAFF initiated salmonella poultry control measures in March 1989, not all were in place until April 1990[7]. It is still too early to draw firm conclusions about the effectiveness of these measures. Meanwhile research continues to investigate the problems surrounding salmonellosis, the nature of the organism, its transmission and appropriate intervention measures. Campylobacter organisms do not often lead to outbreaks of infection. However, careful surveillance has provided evidence that in the spring scavenger birds in some locations contaminate milk delivered to the doorstep. This problem will be addressed in co-operation with the Dairy Industry. The number of cases of listeriosis in England and Wales has declined dramatically over the past two years.

References

1   The Committee on the Microbiological Safety of Food. *The microbiological safety of food: part I: report of the Committee on the Microbiological Safety of Food to the Secretary of State for Health, the Minister of Agriculture, Fisheries and Food, and the Secretaries of State for Wales, Scotland and Northern Ireland.* London: HMSO, 1990. Chairman: Sir Mark Richmond.

2   Department of Health. *Report of the Committee on the Microbiological Safety of Food. Chairman: Sir Mark Richmond. Part I. Recommendations and Government's response.* Heywood (Lancashire): Department of Health, 1990.

Figure 5.6: *Reported cases of listeriosis, 1967-90*

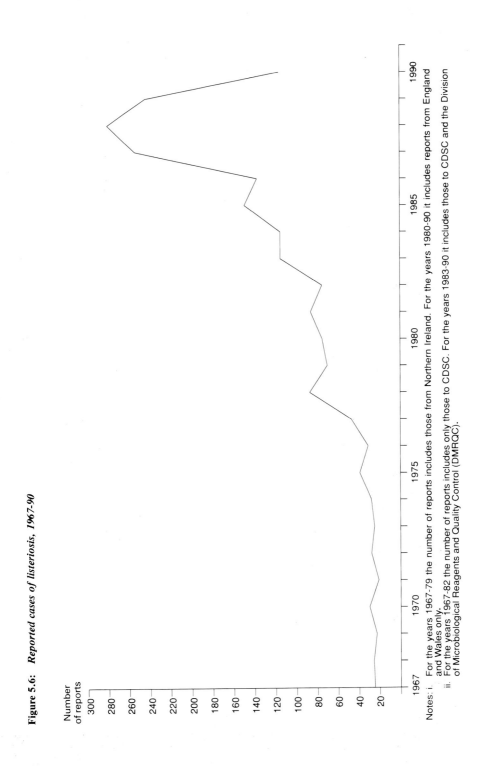

Notes: i. For the years 1967-79 the number of reports includes those from Northern Ireland. For the years 1980-90 it includes reports from England and Wales only.
ii. For the years 1967-82 the number of reports includes only those to CDSC. For the years 1983-90 it includes those to CDSC and the Division of Microbiological Reagents and Quality Control (DMRQC).

133

3   Department of Health. *Food safety efforts cannot be relaxed says Department of Health*. London: Department of Health, 1990. (Press Release 90/506).
4   Hudson SJ, Sobo AO, Russell K, Lightfoot NF. Jackdaws as a potential source of milkborne Campylobacter jejuni infection. *Lancet* 1990; **335**: 1160.
5   Southern JP, Smith R and Palmer SR. Bird attack on milkbottles, a mode of transmission of Campylobacter jejuni to man. *Lancet* 1990; **336**: 1425-7.
6   Department of Health. *Listeria found in pâté*. London: Department of Health, 1989. (Press Release 89/299).
7   *The Zoonoses Order 1988*. London: HMSO, 1989. (SI 1988/2264).

(d) Meningococcal meningitis

The winter upsurge of meningococcal meningitis started earlier than usual in December 1989, and reached higher levels than had been seen in the previous peaks of the present upsurge. It is probable that the influenza epidemic of the winter of 1989 exacerbated the transmission of meningococci and lowered individuals' susceptibility. Following this peak of notifications, levels fell to below those seen in recent years, and, although they rose at the end of the year, notifications were considerably less than in the years immediately prior to 1989. Figure 5.7 shows the 5-week moving averages of meningococcal notifications for England and Wales. There were 1,142 notifications in 1990, compared with 1,139 in 1989 and 1,309 in 1988. Group B strains of meningococci continued to predominate, accounting for approximately 60% of laboratory isolations; Group C strains accounted for around 30%. Laboratory isolations for meningococci during December 1990 were only half those in December 1989.

The Joint Committee on Vaccination and Immunisation (JCVI) considered the epidemiology of *Haemophilus influenzae b* infection in childhood, the availability of conjugate *Haemophilus influenzae b* (Hib) vaccine, and an implementation programme for the incorporation of such a vaccine into the routine childhood schedule. JCVI recommended to the UK Health Departments that Hib vaccine should be introduced, subject to appropriate licensing, in the autumn of 1992. In Finland, where Hib vaccine is in routine use, cases of invasive disease from *Haemophilus influenzae b* are no longer seen in the paediatric wards.

(e) Legionellosis

A provisional total of 179 cases of Legionnaires' disease amongst residents of England and Wales were reported to CDSC in 1990. This is the lowest recorded total since 1984. As in previous years the number of cases in men exceeded that in women by just over 3 to 1 (138 men, 41 women); 20 people (11%) died.

Only 23 cases were associated with outbreaks, compared with 65 in 1989 and 138 in 1988, and there was no major outbreak. Whether this reflects a greater awareness of cooling towers as a potential source of infection, and recognition that good maintenance prevents outbreaks of legionellosis, remains to be seen. Small clusters of three or four cases continued to occur, and ten cases were associated with Chorley Town Centre in September–November.

Half the total number of cases (89) was associated with travel abroad and nine were associated with travel within the UK. It is DH's policy to report these cases back to the local health authority. Where three or more such cases can be associated with the same source, DH endeavours to obtain feedback about the action that has been taken.

Figure 5.7: *5-week moving averages for meningococcal meningitis notifications, England and Wales, 1984 to 22 March 1991*

Numbers

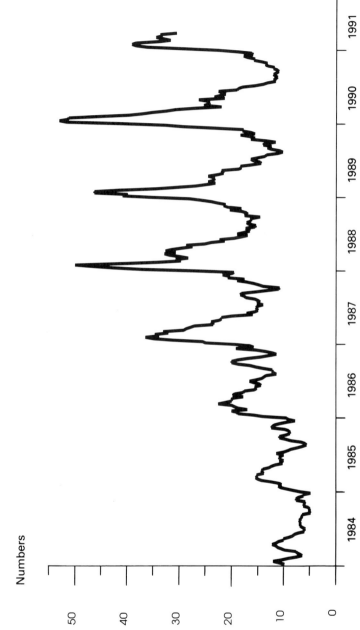

The Joint Health and Safety Executive (HSE) and DH Working Group on Legionellosis will be reporting to the Chief Medical Officer and the Health and Safety Commission early in 1991 on further possible measures to prevent and control legionellosis. The Working Group is likely to stress the importance of good design and proper maintenance procedures in reducing the potential risk of outbreaks associated with building water systems and wet cooling plant. Further research into the epidemiology of sporadic cases is also likely to be recommended in an attempt to identify further ways of reducing the incidence of legionellosis.

(f) Immunisation

Immunisation uptake continues to rise. Polio, diphtheria and tetanus vaccine uptakes in children reaching their second birthday between 1 April 1989 and 31 March 1990 were 89%; measles (or measles, mumps and rubella (MMR)) vaccine uptake was 84%; and pertussis vaccine uptake was 78%. Figure 5.8 shows the national immunisation uptake rates for England for the period 1983 to 1991. Data up to 1 April 1990 are national annual statistics. Data from May 1990 to February 1991 reflect quarterly returns to the COVER programme organised by CDSC, and, as almost all District Health Authorities (DHAs) are submitting quarterly data, these provide excellent proxies for national performance. The most recent measurements show that the national uptake of diphtheria, tetanus and polio vaccines is 90%, and that the 90% national target has been reached for two successive quarters. MMR vaccine uptake continues to rise and is now 89%. Uptake of pertussis vaccine is accelerating.

By 1 April 1990, 51 DHAs had reached or exceeded 90% uptake for measles vaccine, and two DHAs (Oxford and Northallerton) had reached or exceeded 90% uptake for all seven antigens. The February 1991 COVER report shows that, in the preceding quarter, 115 DHAs reached or exceeded the 90% target for measles vaccine, and 36 DHAs achieved this for all seven antigens. Figure 5.9 shows the progressive improvement in DHAs reaching their targets for diphtheria, tetanus, polio and measles vaccine uptakes. Considerable improvements are evident in pertussis vaccine uptake. The following initiatives have contributed to these successes:

- Professional and public information and education campaigns on the benefits and safety of immunisation.

- The extensive use of computer services for call and recall, and for feeding back immunisation performance data to service providers.

- The use of immunisation coverage targets in the health promotion and disease prevention objectives of Regional Health Authorities (RHAs).

- The appointment of immunisation co-ordinators to take responsibility for the immunisation programme in all DHAs.

The data reported here reflect immunisations that were given some considerable time before the date of calculation of uptake. Further improvements can be expected when the results become available for children who were immunised according to the new accelerated schedule (with the primary vaccines given at 2,

Figure 5.8: *Immunisation uptake rate, England, 1983-February 1991*

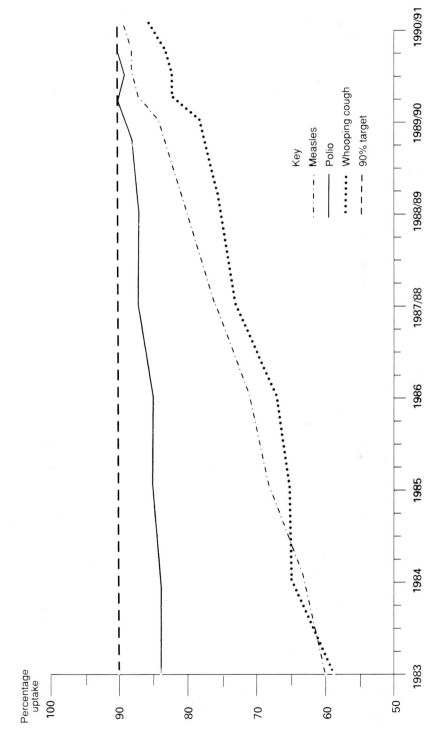

Figure 5.9: *District Health Authorities reaching or exceeding 90% immunisation uptake, England, 1987/88-February 1991*

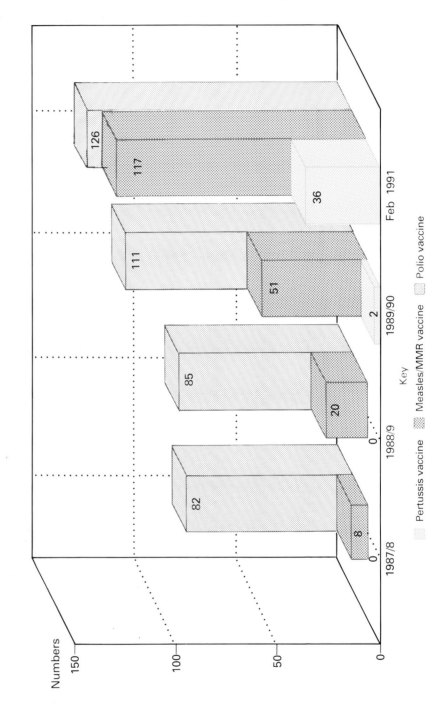

3 and 4 months), and when they fall into cohorts whose uptake is included in the target payment scheme for GPs. The impact of these changes is likely to lift the national immunisation uptake levels to over 90% in even more parts of the country.

Measles, mumps and rubella vaccine—the first two years

The purpose of the policy change

Prior to October 1988, rubella immunisation was recommended for all schoolgirls aged 11–14 years, and women who on screening were found to be rubella susceptible. Despite high uptake of rubella vaccine amongst schoolgirls and low susceptibility amongst ante-natal women, there were still reports of cases of congenital rubella syndrome (CRS) and many rubella infections in pregnancy. It was therefore decided to augment the selective rubella immunisation strategy with the provision of rubella vaccine to young children of both sexes in order to interrupt the transmission of rubella virus, thereby protecting rubella susceptible pregnant women. Further anticipated benefits were an increase in the uptake of measles vaccine, and the elimination of mumps through the use of a combined MMR vaccine, which had been shown to be popular in other countries.

Uptake of measles, mumps and rubella vaccine

Following the introduction of measles vaccine in 1968, uptake rose gradually and reached 76% for the year 1987/88. By that time, only eight DHAs had reached or exceeded 90% uptake. Less than two years after the introduction of MMR vaccine, national uptake in 1989/90 reached 84%, and 51 DHAs had attained or exceeded 90% uptake. Figures 5.10 and 5.11 compare the DHA uptake of measles vaccine in 1987/88 with that of MMR vaccine in 1989/90.

Vaccine supply

It is recommended that MMR vaccine should be given to all children (instead of single antigen measles vaccine) at 12–15 months-of-age, and to older children at the same time as the school entry diphtheria, tetanus and polio booster immunisations. If all of these groups of children had received MMR vaccine, 2.4 million doses would have been required for the first two years. In fact, more than 4 million doses were distributed to health authorities over the first two years, suggesting that not only have the selected children been immunised, but also that many of those in between the recommended ages, and some older children, have received MMR vaccine.

Impact on rubella

Rubella was not a notifiable disease before October 1988, although detailed rubella surveillance was undertaken in other ways. Figure 5.12 shows the rates of monthly reports of rubella from the Royal College of General Practitioners' (RCGP's) Sentinel practices. Clinical reporting of rubella infections is notoriously unreliable but, nevertheless, a considerable decrease in the number of cases can be seen. Surveillance of laboratory reports of rubella infections in pregnant women and children under the age of 15 years has demonstrated a

Figure 5.10: *Measles vaccine uptake by the age of 2 years. England, 1987/88*

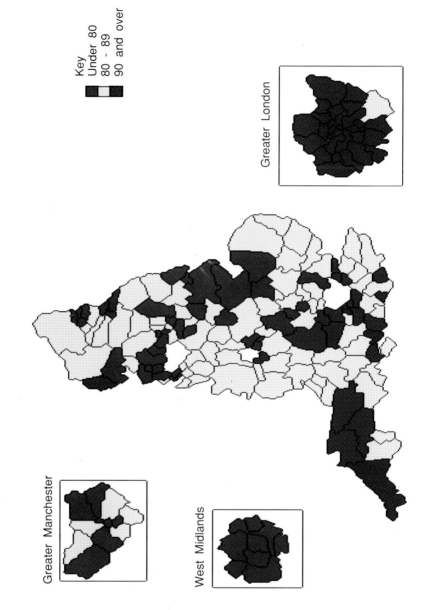

Key
Under 80
80 - 89
90 and over

Greater London

Greater Manchester

West Midlands

140

Figure 5.11: *Measles vaccine uptake by the age of 2 years, England, 1989/90*

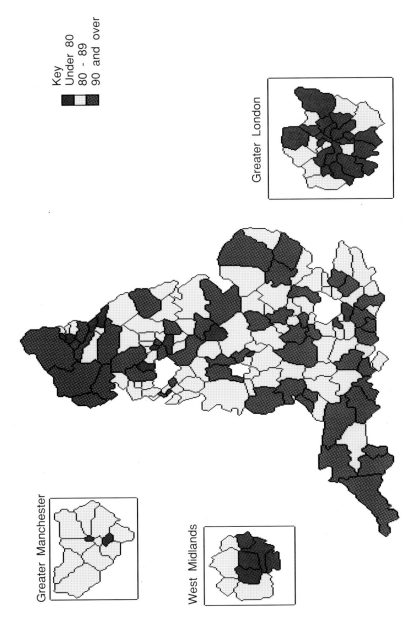

Key
Under 80
80 - 89
90 and over

Greater London

Greater Manchester

West Midlands

141

Figure 5.12: *4-weekly reports of rubella from the RCGP's Sentinel practices, England and Wales, 1985-January 1991*

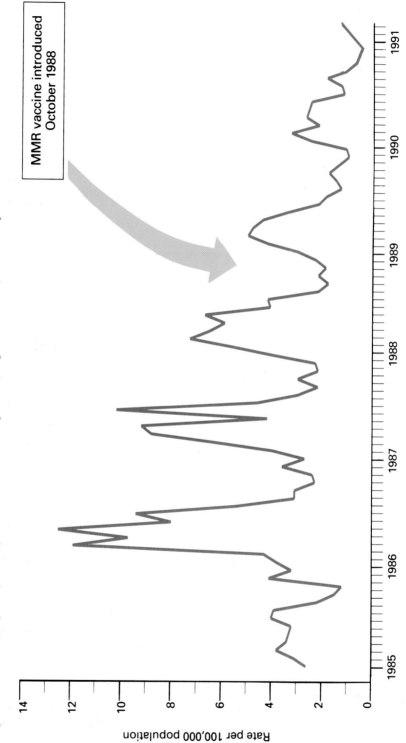

Figure 5.13: *Notification of measles, England and Wales, 1940-90*

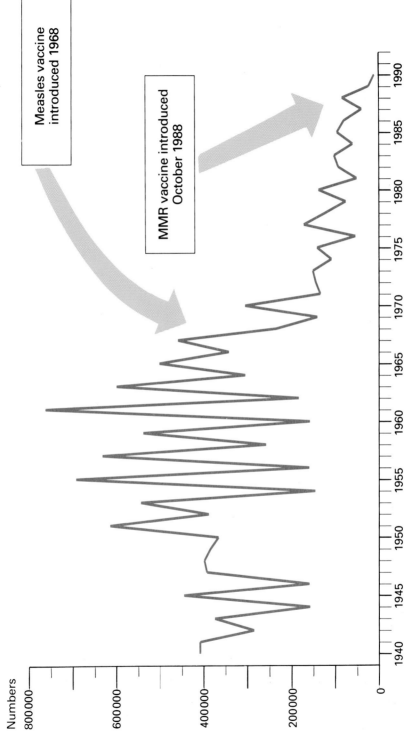

143

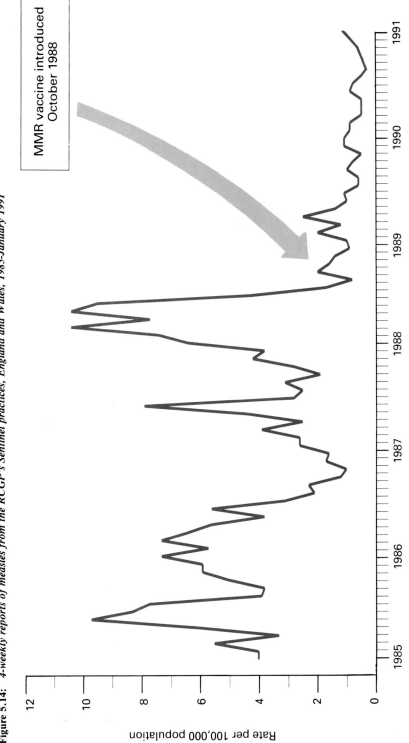

Figure 5.14: *4-weekly reports of measles from the RCGP's Sentinel practices, England and Wales, 1985-January 1991*

144

Figure 5.15: *4-weekly reports of mumps from the RCGP's Sentinel practices, England and Wales, 1985-January 1991*

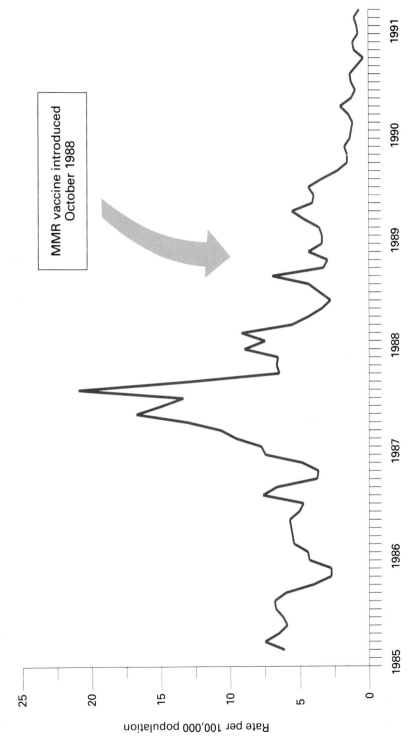

MMR vaccine introduced
October 1988

Rate per 100,000 population

close correlation between upsurges of rubella in such children and infections in pregnant women. The number of laboratory confirmed rubella infections in both groups has fallen dramatically since the introduction of MMR vaccine.

Impact on measles

In the past, despite measles immunisation, epidemics of measles have occurred approximately every other year, with 100,000 or more notified cases during epidemic years. In 1989, there were 26,180 notifications, the lowest number ever. Although 1990 was expected to be an epidemic year, notifications halved again to 13,291, with matching decreases in morbidity and mortality. During that year not one death from acute measles in England and Wales was reported to OPCS. This is the first year that children have not died of acute measles since records began. Figure 5.13 shows the annual notifications for measles for England and Wales for the period 1940 to 1990; the impact of the introduction of MMR vaccine is evident. Figure 5.14, derived from data from the RCGP's Sentinel practices, confirms the near disappearance of measles.

Impact on mumps

In the past, mumps led to between 1,200 and 1,500 hospital admissions each year, mostly following the development of meningitis or encephalitis. Mumps became notifiable only in October 1988, and since then notifications have fallen progressively to approximately 50 per week for England and Wales. Mumps was previously reported by the RCGP's Sentinel practices, and Figure 5.15 shows the dramatic decline in mumps reporting since the introduction of MMR vaccine.

Conclusion

In the space of two years, MMR vaccine has had a dramatic impact on all three target diseases. CRS, with its potentially devastating impact on the fetus, has been almost eliminated, and rubella infections in pregnant women, which previously led to cases of CRS or terminations of pregnancy, are lower than ever before. Notifications of measles have been reduced by 90% and mumps is close to elimination. Despite these successes, there are no grounds for complacency. If measles is to be eliminated, even higher levels of immunisation uptake are required in every locality. Any pockets of low uptake will allow accumulation of susceptible individuals amongst whom measles epidemics will undoubtedly occur.

(g) Influenza

By the beginning of 1990 the influenza epidemic of late 1989 had already peaked, and influenza levels had fallen to those usually seen at that time of the year. In the latter part of 1990 influenza activity was at a low level, and most isolates were of influenza B.

Investigation of the causes of the excess mortality which occurred during the epidemic of 1989/90, and which was described in the Report for 1989[1], was undertaken. There were almost 30,000 excess deaths in Great Britain during the 55 days of the epidemic, reaching a peak 29 days after its start. There were

11,000 fewer deaths than expected during the three months following the epidemic, suggesting that the majority of deaths during the epidemic were not of people who would have been likely to die within three months. Over 80% of the excess deaths were in people aged 75 years or over, and 43% were in people aged over 85 years. Although only 10% of the deaths were ascribed to influenza on the death certificate, nearly half were due to respiratory causes. There was also a significant rise in mortality from cardiovascular disease, in those with mental conditions, and possibly among those with endocrine conditions, principally diabetes.

In the months leading up to the epidemic, influenza vaccination had again been recommended for those at special risk of developing complications from influenza[2], ie those, particularly the elderly, with chronic cardiac and pulmonary disease, chronic renal failure, diabetes mellitus and immunosuppression, and elderly persons living in residential homes and long-stay accommodation. Although over 3 million doses were given, it is far from clear to what extent the recommended policy was implemented.

References

1   Department of Health. *On the State of the Public Health: the annual report of the Chief Medical Officer of the Department of Health for the year 1989*. London: HMSO, 1990; 8.
2   Department of Health. *Influenza*. London: Department of Health, 1990. (Professional Letter: PL/CMO(90)9).

(h) Cryptosporidiosis

Following an outbreak of cryptosporidiosis in Swindon and Oxfordshire in early 1989, the Minister for Water, in consultation with DH, set up an Expert Group under the chairmanship of Sir John Badenoch to advise the Government on the significance of cryptosporidium in water supplies. The Report of the Expert Group was published in July 1990[1]. The Government accepted all 51 recommendations, and measures have already been taken to implement those for which DH is responsible. In particular, efforts have been made to ensure that all health authorities have established links with their local water companies and have, in conjunction with them and the local authority, formulated an outbreak control plan which comes into operation if a waterborne outbreak of cryptosporidiosis occurs in their locality. It is anticipated that the plan could also be used for all water-borne outbreaks of illness which are microbiological in origin.

In addition, in 1991 the Department will be organising a series of seminars on the *Public Health Aspects of Drinking Water Supplies—A Microbiological Prospective*. They will be held Regionally and be specifically targeted at newly appointed Directors of Public Health (DsPH) and Consultants in Communicable Disease Control (CsCDC). It is hoped that the seminars will provide a useful base of knowledge and foster greater liaison between colleagues in the water industry and health authorities.

Reference

1   Group of experts on cryptosporidium in water supplies, Department of Health, Department of the Environment. *Cryptosporidium in water supplies: report of the group of experts*. London: HMSO, 1990. Chairman: Sir John Badenoch.

(i) Viral hepatitis

Although hepatitis may occur in the course of a large number of viral infections, the term 'viral hepatitis' refers to those infections in which the liver is the major site of organ damage. The viruses responsible are a heterogeneous group of organisms, varying not only in their physical characteristics, but also in their routes of transmission, pathogenicity and natural history of infection.

Viral hepatitis is a notifiable disease. In 1990, a provisional total of 9,005 cases was notified to OPCS from England and Wales, an increase of over 25% in comparison with the previous year (see Figure 5.16). Since 1987 notifications to OPCS have been categorised as hepatitis A, hepatitis B, hepatitis non-A non-B, and hepatitis other/not known. Although one form of hepatitis non-A non-B has been characterised as hepatitis C, reliable tests for use on a routine basis are only now becoming available, and specific epidemiological data are not yet being collected. Another source of data on incidence is the laboratory reporting of acute hepatitis A and B in England to CDSC (see Figures 5.17 and 5.18).

Hepatitis A

Hepatitis A is transmitted by the faeco-oral route and is endemic in many parts of the world. At present there is no licensed vaccine to confer active protection, but passive protection, using human immunoglobulin, is offered to family contacts and those travelling to areas of high prevalence. It is also used during outbreaks of the infection.

Endemic hepatitis A occurs wherever hygienic standards are low. As these improve, transmission becomes intermittent. The most recent peak year for hepatitis A was 1982, when there were 4,091 cases reported to CDSC from England. The reported incidence has increased in each of the past four years as shown in Figures 5.16 and 5.17. In 1990, the provisional number of reports of cases of acute hepatitis A in England received by CDSC was 7,214, compared with 5,061 reports in 1989. In 1989, 7,071 cases of viral hepatitis were reported to OPCS, of which 5,278 were hepatitis A. The provisional data for 1990 indicate that the total number of reports rose to 9,005, of which 7,316 were reports of hepatitis A. There has been an increase in reports from most Regions, but particularly from some Regions in the North of England; the increased incidence can also be attributed to clusters of outbreaks in certain towns and cities. As prevalence of the virus declines, outbreaks are likely to involve more people because of low levels of immunity within the general population. Only an active vaccine is likely to alter this.

Figure 5.16: *Quarterly reports of hepatitis A and hepatitis B to OPCS, England and Wales, 1987-90*

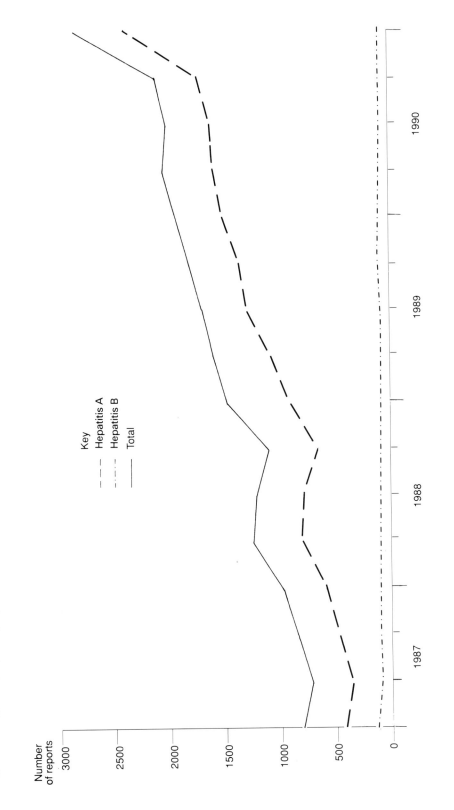

Figure 5.17: *Annual reports of hepatitis A to CDSC, England, 1980-90*

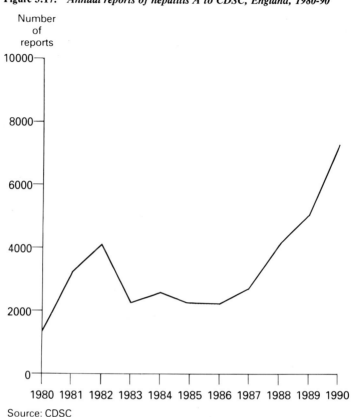

Source: CDSC

Hepatitis B

In 1990, a provisional total of 526 cases of acute hepatitis B was reported to CDSC from England. The incidence of hepatitis B peaked in 1984; it has been declining since then, although the rate of decline in the last three years has been low. Figure 5.18 shows the incidence since 1980.

Those belonging to high-risk groups in whom vaccination against hepatitis B should be considered are listed in *Immunisation against Infectious Disease*, a new edition of which was published in 1990[1]. Between 1985 and 1990 the incidence of acute hepatitis B declined in most of the risk groups, as shown in Table 5.11. This decline may, in part, be attributable to vaccination policy, particularly among occupational risk groups. Behavioural change, as a result of the public education campaigns about HIV infection and AIDS, may account for much of the decline in some other risk groups, although the increased incidence seen in some groups in 1990 may be linked to a failure to maintain this behavioural change.

Reference

1 Department of Health, Welsh Office, Scottish Home and Health Department. *Immunisation against infectious disease.* London: HMSO, 1990.

Figure 5.18: *Annual reports of hepatitis B to CDSC, England, 1980-90*

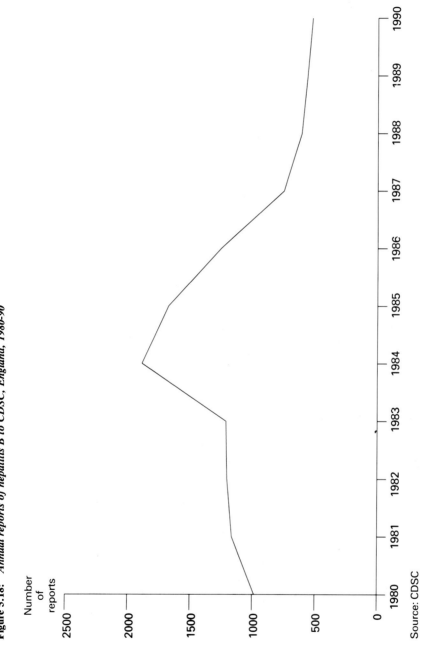

Source: CDSC

Table 5.11: *Incidence of acute hepatitis B in selected risk groups, England, 1985-90*

History	Number of patients						Total
	1985	1986	1987	1988	1989	1990	
Injecting drug misuse	502	283	144	104	67	82	1182
Homosexual/bisexual male	121	106	50	47	40	76	440
Contact with a case or carrier	166	134	76	51	26	48	501
Transfusion	7	8	12	16	10	14	67
Bleeding disorder	7	3	4	2	0	0	16
Patients in institutions for the mentally handicapped	5	8	9	5	3	4	34
Health care staff	43	34	26	20	16	12	151
Others/Not stated	828	682	431	367	404	290	3002
Total	1679	1258	752	612	566	526	5393

Source: CDSC (unpublished)

(j) Tuberculosis

Between 1982 and 1987, total notifications of tuberculosis in England and Wales fell from 7,410 to 5,086. In 1988, notifications increased by 1.5% compared with 1987, and in 1989 they increased by 5.2% compared with 1988. The total for 1990 is 4.2% less than that for 1989, although it is still 0.7% higher than that for 1988 (see Figure 5.19).

These figures have been followed closely because of the findings in the USA, where a progressive fall in notifications of tuberculosis over 30 years has been reversed since 1984, and the reversal has been attributed to the epidemic of infection with HIV.

In England and Wales, the highest rates of tuberculosis are in people whose ethnic origin is the Indian subcontinent. In other groups, the highest rates are in those aged over 65 years. The lowest rates are in the young white population. In contrast, the majority of patients with HIV infection or AIDS are young white males. Thus the overlap between these two groups is small. Tuberculosis has been diagnosed in about 4% of people with AIDS in the UK, and other mycobacterial infections in a further 4% of cases. Despite the likelihood that these cases are under-reported, they are unlikely to have been responsible for the recent changes in the notification rates for tuberculosis. Further detailed monitoring is essential to assess the impact of the HIV epidemic on the incidence of tuberculosis in this country.

Schools BCG programme

In 1990, JCVI decided that, until more is known of the likely impact of the HIV epidemic on the incidence of tuberculosis in this country, the schools BCG programme should continue. This decision will be reviewed in the mid-1990s. Supplies of BCG vaccine have now been restored.

Figure 5.19: *Tuberculosis in England and Wales, 1982-90*

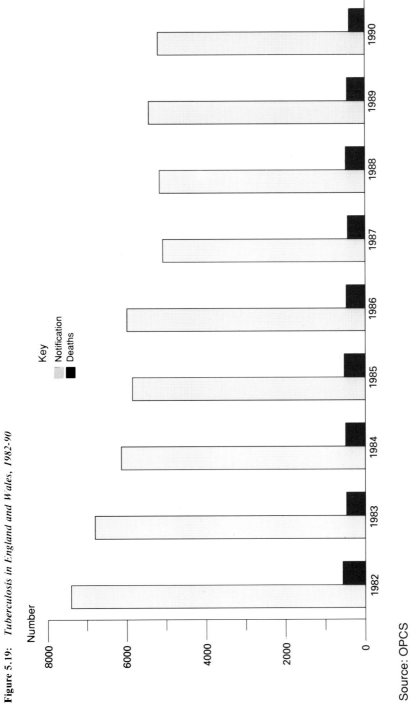

Source: OPCS

153

(k) Bovine spongiform encephalopathy

Increasing numbers of cases of this disease in British cattle were reported in 1990, with a cumulative total of nearly 22,000 confirmed cases by the end of the year. In spite of much speculation by the media, there is no evidence that this disease has been, or is expected to be, a risk to human health. Nevertheless, following advice from independent experts, initially a committee under the chairmanship of Sir Richard Southwood, and more recently a committee under the chairmanship of Dr David Tyrrell, various actions have been taken to reduce human exposure to infected or potentially infected bovine material.

In May 1990, following the first description of a spongiform encephalopathy in a cat, and anxieties expressed by a number of our European partners, the safety of British beef was questioned by the media. The advice from the Tyrrell committee was reassuring. They concluded that beef could be eaten safely by everyone. Even in the unlikely event that the virulence of the bovine spongiform encephalopathy (BSE) agent was different from that of scrapie, if there were any hazard for man from oral ingestion of beef or beef products, the risk would be very small indeed. To allay public concern a statement to that effect was issued by the Chief Medical Officer on 15 May. Subsequently the Agriculture Select Committee[1], in reporting on BSE, agreed that the scientific evidence supported the safety of beef from British herds. The Committee condemned the irresponsible activity of the media and others for arousing fears on ill-founded speculation.

Monitoring of all UK cases of Creutzfeldt-Jakob Disease (CJD) began in 1990. In spite of the publicity which might have been expected to increase ascertainment of this rare disorder, the incidence of confirmed cases of CJD appears unchanged from that in the early 1980s, the last occasion on which such a study took place[2].

References

1   House of Commons Agriculture Committee. *Bovine Spongiform Encephalopathy (BSE): fifth report of the Agriculture Committee, session 1989-90: report and proceedings of the Committee, together with minutes of evidence and appendices.* London: HMSO, 1990.
2   Harries-Jones R, Knight R, Will R, Cousens S, Smith P, Mathews W. Creutzfeldt-Jakob disease in England and Wales, 1980-1984: a case control study of potential risk factors. *J Neurol Neurosurg Psychiatry* 1988; **51:** 1113-9.

6. THE NATIONAL HEALTH SERVICE AND COMMUNITY CARE REFORMS

(a) Implementation of the National Health Service reforms

The White Paper, *Working for Patients*[1], was published at the end of January 1989. The necessary legal framework for realising its proposals was contained in the National Health Service and Community Care Act 1990[2], which received Royal Assent on 29 June 1990. However, practical preparations for the reforms were made throughout 1990, taking the form of a structured implementation programme agreed between the National Health Service (NHS) and the NHS Management Executive (ME).

The programme provided the opportunity for close joint working between the NHS and the ME. The ME promoted and supported a great deal of development work in the NHS, with the objective of identifying the best way of putting the reforms into effect; joint working allowed the resolution of issues as they arose. The ME emphasised that the changes needed to introduce the reforms had to be properly managed to ensure a smooth transition. Any changes in patient flows required full assessment and careful management, whilst purchasers and providers were involved in extensive discussion over their respective plans. The objective was to have the basic reforms in place by 1 April 1991, whilst allowing further refinement in the future.

Funding health authorities

Working for Patients[1] proposed a fundamental change in the way the Hospital and Community Health Services are funded, and implementation of the change began in the 1990/91 financial year. Allocations to Regional Health Authorities (RHAs) were based on each Region's resident population, and they were expected to pay for the treatment of their residents in other Regions. Agreed adjustments for these cross boundary flows were made centrally at the start of the year. 1990/91 saw the first step towards funding RHAs on the basis of a new, simpler weighted capitation formula, which mainly reflects the age distribution and relative health of each Region's population. In addition, the Thames Regions had their allocations increased by between 1% and 3% to reflect the higher costs of, and demands on, services in London in particular.

From April 1991, District Health Authorities (DHAs) will also be funded for their resident populations. They will enter into contracts with those hospitals or community health units which can best provide the quality, quantity and range of services their patients need. DHAs will then pay hospitals and community units directly for services provided to their residents. In 1991/92, all Districts will be funded broadly on the basis of the resources currently used by their resident populations. Ultimately, they will be funded on the basis of their weighted populations, and Regions have been asked to make a start in 1991/92 towards District allocations made on this basis. Since the circumstances of Districts vary more than those of Regions, allocations to Districts may need to be rather more sensitive to local factors than those to Regions. The use of additional weighting factors at this level, for instance to reflect variations in social deprivation, is under consideration.

The new structures and functions of health authorities and Family Health Services Authorities

Under the new Act[2] RHAs were reconstituted on 26 July 1990; DHAs, Family Health Services Authorities (FHSAs) and London Postgraduate Special Hospital Authorities (SHAs) were reconstituted on 17 September 1990; the smaller membership enables authorities to strengthen their corporate role as management bodies providing a focus for effective decision making.

RHAs now comprise a chairman and five non-executive members (including an FHSA Chairman and a representative of a university with a medical or dental school) appointed by the Secretary of State, and up to five executive members. The general manager/chief executive and the chief finance officer are appointed as executive members ex-officio; other executive members are appointed by the Chairman, the non-executive members and the general manager/chief executive. RHAs' principal functions include the co-ordination of purchasing policy, allocation of resources and monitoring of performance.

DHAs also have a chairman, five non-executive members and up to five executive members. There is no requirement for an FHSA Chairman to be a non-executive member of a DHA, or for a university representative unless it is a teaching District. The Chairman is appointed by the Secretary of State, and the non-executive members by the RHA. The general manager and the chief finance officer are ex-officio members. DHAs assess the health needs of their populations, purchase potentially cost-effective and appropriate services for them, and evaluate the outcomes of those services in terms of health gains; they also have the responsibility for managing the contracts that they place. In addition to their purchasing function, DHAs retain an overall responsibility to improve the health of their populations. As part of this wider remit they are responsible for the prevention, surveillance and control of communicable disease, and the provision of public health medicine advice to local authorities, FHSAs and others within their geographical boundaries.

During 1990, DHAs established purchasing teams (including Directors of Public Health (DsPH)) to prepare contracts for 1991/92 based on the services currently provided to District residents. This process was supported by the ME's DHA project, which has been working with a group of health authorities to develop the new role. A number of important papers have been published to provide advice, including the means to relate needs assessment to contracting. To facilitate this work, a programme of research reviews has been established to make the results of epidemiological studies more accessible to DHAs.

FHSAs comprise a chairman appointed by the Secretary of State, nine non-executive members appointed by the RHA, including a general practitioner (GP), a dentist, a pharmacist, a nurse with experience of managing community services (all of whom serve in a personal, rather than a representative capacity) and five lay members, and the general manager as an ex-officio member. FHSAs work closely with DHAs and have responsibilities for assessing local population needs for family health services, planning and developing services to meet those needs, and managing the contracts of family practitioners, including the targeting of cash-limited funds for general medical practitioners' ancillary staff and premises to areas of greatest need.

The London Postgraduate SHAs have a chairman and six non-executive members appointed by the Secretary of State. Up to six executive members may be appointed, and they must include the general manager/chief executive, the chief finance officer (both of whom are ex-officio), a medical director and a nursing director. However, the Eastman Dental SHA has only five executive members who must include the general manager/chief executive, the chief finance officer and a dental director.

National Health Service Trusts

NHS Trusts are a key element of the NHS and community care reforms. By the end of January 1991, 57 hospitals and other units had been approved for Trust status; they will become fully operational from 1 April 1991. A further 123 hospitals and units have expressed an interest in becoming Trusts from 1 April 1992.

In order to assure a significant measure of operational independence, Trusts have the freedom to:

- acquire, own and dispose of assets to ensure the most effective use is made of them;

- make their own cases for capital developments directly to the NHS ME;

- borrow money, within annually agreed limits, primarily for building and equipment, and for upgrading existing buildings;

- create their own management structures;

- employ their own staff, determine their own staffing structures, and set their own terms and conditions of employment (with the exceptions that junior doctors in training will continue to have national pay and conditions of service, and that the contracts of employment for registrars and senior registrars will continue to be held and administered by RHAs); and

- advertise their services, within guidelines set down by professional codes of practice on such advertising.

Contracting for National Health Service services

The introduction of contracts provides the mechanism through which funds are passed from those purchasing health services to those providing them. The need to secure funding will encourage all units to provide high quality, consumer responsive services. Contracts will also enable purchasers to specify and monitor the nature and quality of services their residents or patients receive.

The ME is monitoring the introduction of contracting to ensure a smooth transition into the new system with no disruption to patient services. The evidence is that most purchasers are seeking to secure block contracts which maintain existing patient flows, except where change is planned and managed. These arrangements, similar to current practice, will maintain stability, but will allow the contracting process to evolve and grow in sophistication over time.

During 1990 there was extensive consultation between DHAs and local GPs to ensure that the former secure contracts with the providers to whom GPs prefer to send their patients. It seems that the majority of GPs are more interested in securing high quality services from their traditional providers than seeking to change their referral patterns. There was also consultation with clinicians and other professional staff on service specifications. Clinicians provided valuable advice on whether the terms of contracts are both realistic and deliverable.

The information systems needed to support more sophisticated contracting are not yet generally available. Nevertheless, purchasers and providers are specifying in contracts quality terms which are both challenging and achievable. These range from specifying the maximum waiting times for inpatient and outpatient appointments to conducting regular consumer satisfaction surveys among patients.

The Localities Project

The Localities Project is a large-scale development project lasting 2-3 years and involving six NHS sites. Its aim is to address the overall impact of the reforms by enabling the sites, who made good progress in preparing for the new arrangements, to implement the reforms to a greater degree of sophistication more quickly than elsewhere in the NHS. In December 1990, after a selection process in which 23 bids were entered by the 14 Regions, the following sites based on DHA areas were chosen by the ME:

Cornwall
Halton, St Helens and Knowsley and Warrington
Newcastle
Portsmouth and South East Hampshire
Wandsworth
West Dorset

They show a wide range of characteristics and face different issues and problems. All, however, will be expected to work on issues common to the NHS as a whole, while also concentrating on issues more specific to themselves. For example, Newcastle will be examining Service Increment for Teaching and Research (SIFTR) issues, and the Mersey DHAs will be considering the implications of consortium arrangements in delivering the reforms.

Contracts running from January 1991 to March 1992 were agreed with the sites. The format—a common core of issues and tasks—was designed to ensure a framework of co-operation and collaboration to a common overall purpose. The contracts also offer flexibility to encompass local initiatives and to take full advantage of the diversity offered by the wide range of sites participating in the project. Feedback on tackling various issues in advance of most of the rest of the NHS will keep the ME closely informed of progress with the reforms, while at the same time providing the rest of the NHS with practical lessons on how to tackle problems of implementation, and demonstrating what can be achieved under the new arrangements.

GP fundholding scheme

Under the fundholding scheme, general practices will be given funds to cover three key areas of health expenditure: certain hospital services, prescribing costs and part of practice staff costs. Fundholders will be able to move money between these three elements. The scheme will enable GPs to make decisions about how NHS money can best be used to meet the needs of their patients. They will be able to use monies saved at the end of the year on any service or facility that will benefit their patients.

In December 1989, the Department of Health (DH) issued details of the scheme to all GPs[3]. Although over 850 practices initially registered interest in the scheme, not all were eligible to join and some decided to defer participation until the second year. Nevertheless, during 1990, over 300 practices commenced the preparatory work necessary to become fundholders. This included the collection of data on referral and treatment patterns for the hospital procedures covered by the scheme, and discussions with provider units on costing and quality issues. Such information was required by RHAs in order to determine the hospital element of the fund.

During the year the Department also provided guidance on various issues associated with fundholding, including contracting by fundholding practices, financial issues, the scope of the fund, and a Manual of Accounts dealing with technical issues surrounding the accounting procedures to be followed[4]. In addition the Department contracted with accountants experienced in the work of GPs to provide a telephone helpline to deal with any queries on the Manual.

In August 1990, the major computer suppliers to GPs started work on production of the specialised software which practices will use to keep track of the use made of their fund. Conformance testing of the software started in December, with training on its use being provided by the companies involved. The Department introduced a reimbursement scheme to meet the full cost of the software. In addition, some practices realised that they would require additional computer hardware; a sliding scale reimbursement scheme was introduced to assist them to meet the costs incurred.

RHAs, FHSAs and practices have all been closely involved in the implementation of the scheme. FHSAs have the responsibility to monitor practices to ensure that the fund is managed properly, and adequate patient care provided. The effect on patient care will also be carefully assessed by DH and independent researchers.

Indicative Prescribing Scheme

The Indicative Prescribing Scheme was first described in *Working for Patients: Working Paper 4*[5] and elaborated in May 1990 in *Improving Prescribing*[6]. The thrust of this initiative is to reduce wasteful prescribing, of which there is much evidence. The wide variation in cost from area to area, the quantities of returned medications, and the rising cost of prescriptions beyond general inflation all pointed to the need for an initiative which would, through education, support an element of increased financial rigour and check any excessive prescribing. Under the scheme each practice will be allocated an indicative amount for prescribed medicines annually; it should only be exceeded 'with good cause'. The amount will be set by the FHSA on specialist medical advice, and take full account of the needs of the practice. Allowance will be made for inflationary pressures. GPs will be supported by enhanced information systems, medical advice from specialist advisers appointed by each FHSA, and education in the form of drug Bulletins from the Departmentally funded Medicines Resource Centre. The advisers themselves will be provided with continuing education from the new Medical Advisers Support Centre. Research into the quality of prescribing and the information systems by the Prescribing Research Unit at Leeds University has already begun.

Quality of care

Central to the NHS reforms is the Government's commitment to improve the quality of care. There was a great deal of work on quality throughout the NHS in 1990, building on the centrally funded initiatives started in 1989/90. In 1990/91 £10 million was made available, of which £7.5 million was allocated directly to Regions to fund their own local quality initiatives. The remaining £2.5 million was used to fund a national quality exhibition at the Birmingham NEC, national demonstration projects in Total Quality Management, Outpatient Departments and Accident and Emergency Departments, and other quality initiatives.

Valuable lessons are now beginning to emerge from the first wave of Outpatient Department and Total Quality Management projects, and are being shared with the rest of the NHS. *Demonstrably Different*, a brochure reporting on the first six Outpatient Department demonstration projects, was distributed to health service managers[7]. In 1991/92, £4.2 million will be made available to give further support to the Total Quality Management and Accident and Emergency Department initiatives, and to take forward projects in day case units and primary health care.

Medical audit

The medical focus for improving the quality of care is the audit initiative announced in the NHS review. All doctors who work in primary health care or in hospitals will be expected to participate in a medical audit programme. Medical audit should not be seen as a disciplinary process, but as a method of improving the quality of clinical care. Doctors should take a critical look at their own strengths and weaknesses within a supportive environment and with the help of their peers[8].

During 1990, a structure for developing medical audit was developed in most health authorities. This was made possible by the willing support of the medical profession. All the medical Royal Colleges and Faculties established units to develop methods of audit for use in their own specialties. They are defining standards, agreeing protocols and defining ways of measuring health that can be used in local peer review. This move towards groups of doctors taking a corporate responsibility for the way in which they manage patients and resources will improve the quality of care delivered by the NHS. The measures taken to introduce medical audit in the family health services are described in Chapter 7.

Resource management

The ME continued to make good progress with the implementation of resource management in 1990. A further 155 large acute hospitals entered the national programme during the course of the year. There are now 211 hospitals involved in the resource management programme, representing over 75% of all large acute hospitals in the country. The ME remains on target to meet the *Working for Patients*[1] commitment to have all large acute hospitals involved in resource management by the end of 1991/92.

The Government demonstrated its commitment to resource management by investing over £100 million by the end of 1990/91, with a further £92 million planned for 1991/92. Approximately half is being invested in new information technology systems in every acute hospital. The remainder of the investment will allow hospitals to run a 3-year project to implement resource management, including the retraining of clinicians and managers.

The ME's Resource Management Unit (RMU) offered strong support to hospitals involved in implementing resource management throughout 1990. Support is increasingly being channelled through Regional Resource Management Co-ordinators as RHAs assume a wider role in the resource management programme. A considerable amount of guidance designed for hospital use was prepared by the Unit during the year. It included guidance on resource management nursing information systems; a computer-based training package to help improve clinical coding; and guidance on the role of the resource management project manager. The RMU sponsored a number of resource and development projects to look at the extension of resource management beyond the acute hospital sector, including the role of resource management in small hospitals, Accident and Emergency Departments, and Outpatient Departments. Major conferences were held on resource management in mental health and in the community.

The ME met the Joint Consultants Committee in March 1990 to discuss the involvement of clinicians in hospital management. The Central Consultants and Specialists Committee (CCSC) subsequently issued its own guidance on clinical directorates.

Management training for consultants

During 1990/91 over £1 million was provided for 102 consultants from seven Regions to attend residential management development courses in a pilot programme. The aim was to develop the management skills of consultants, and to help them fulfil their potential in the enhanced role envisaged by the greater delegation of management in both directly managed units and Trusts. Lancaster University will evaluate this pilot scheme in 1991. In 1991/92, the Government will make a further £2.12 million available to extend this scheme. This should enable all Regions to participate, and provide training for around 270 further consultants.

Consultants' contracts and job plans

The Health Departments completed discussions in the first half of 1990 with representatives of the CCSC on the Government's proposals concerning consultants' contracts contained in *Working for Patients: Working Paper 7*[9]. Subsequently, DH advised RHAs to devolve at least to District level the day-to-day management of hospital consultants' contracts. In addition, all hospital consultants should, from 1 April 1991, have a job plan agreed with the manager responsible for the management of the contract. The job plan should cover the main duties and responsibilities of the post, and must include a work programme setting out fixed commitments[10]. Changes were also made to the disciplinary procedures for medical and dental staff[11], to consultants' appointments procedures[12], and to the distinction awards system[13].

References

1 Department of Health. *Working for Patients: the NHS review.* London: HMSO, 1989. (Cm. 555).

2 *National Health Service and Community Care Act 1990.* London: HMSO, 1990.

3 Department of Health. *Practice funding scheme: issue of programme to GPs.* London: Department of Health, 1989. (Executive Letter: EL(89)P199; FPCL 266/89).

4 Department of Health and Central Office of Information. *A guide to General Practice Funding Accounts Systems.* London: Department of Health, 1990.

5 Department of Health. *Working for Patients: Working Paper 4: Indicative Prescribing Budgets for General Medical Practitioners.* London: HMSO, 1989.

6 Department of Health. *Improving Prescribing: the implementation of the GP Indicative Prescribing Scheme.* Heywood (Lancashire): Department of Health, 1990.

7 Department of Health: NHS Management Executive. *Demonstrably different.* London: Department of Health, 1991.

8 Berwick DM. Continuous improvement as an ideal in health care. *N Engl J Med* 1989; **320**(1):53-6.

9 Department of Health. *Working for Patients: Working Paper 7: NHS consultants: appointments, contracts and distinction awards.* London: HMSO, 1989.

10 Department of Health. *Consultants contracts and job plans.* Heywood (Lancashire): Department of Health, 1990. (Health Circular: HC(90)16).

11 Department of Health. *Disciplinary procedures for hospital and community medical and dental staff.* Heywood (Lancashire): Department of Health, 1990. (Health Circular: HC(90)9).

12 Department of Health. *Health services management: the appointment of consultants and directors of public health.* Heywood (Lancashire): Department of Health, 1990. (Health Circular: HC(90)19).

13 Department of Health. *Pay and conditions of service: distinction awards.* London: Department of Health, 1990. (Executive Letter EL(90)141).

(b) Implementation of the community care reforms

The Government's plans for the development of community care were set out in the White Paper, *Caring for People: Community Care in the Next Decade and Beyond*[1]. The necessary legislation has been put in place by the National Health Service and Community Care Act 1990[2]. Implementation of the new arrangements for care in the community will go ahead on a phased timetable leading to full implementation of the policy in April 1993. The overriding objective of the reforms is to enable people to live independently in the community for as long as they are able and wish to do so. The timetable for introducing the reforms is:

April 1991:

Introduction of new inspection units and complaints procedures within local authorities. Two Specific Grants for mental illness and drug and alcohol services will become available.

April 1992:

Local authorities will produce and publish their community care plans jointly with DHAs and FHSAs. These plans will show the planning agreements reached between agencies, particularly at the interface of health and social care.

April 1993:

Full implementation of the new system. Assessment procedures will be introduced, and local authorities will assume responsibility for assessing the needs of clients both for support at home as well as for residential and nursing home care. The 'care' element of funds currently held by the Department of Social Security will be transferred.

Many of the procedures which local authorities will be implementing correspond to similar procedures being introduced within the NHS. Local authorities will increasingly act as enablers and commissioners of services, basing their purchase of services on an assessment of their populations' needs for social care. The assessment of population needs for health care undertaken by DsPH is likely to include information which local authorities will find valuable in making their assessments of the need for social care.

It is essential that GPs and other doctors are adequately involved in individual assessments for community care, in order to ensure that health care needs receive the attention they deserve. The key to making a successful reality of community care is partnership between agencies at local level, maximising the effect of all the resources available in the community.

DH has issued policy guidance to local and health authorities[3]. This guidance was developed as a result of wide-ranging consultation with statutory agencies, the voluntary and private sectors, and with professionals in both the health and social care fields. Practice material is being developed by the Social Services Inspectorate (SSI) in partnership with local and health authorities, and is being published throughout the implementation timetable. Progress towards implementation is being monitored by the SSI and RHAs.

References

1   Department of Health. *Caring for People: community care in the next decade and beyond.* London: HMSO, 1989. (Cm. 849).
2   *National Health Service and Community Care Act 1990.* London: HMSO, 1990.
3   Department of Health. *Caring for People: community care in the next decade and beyond: policy guidance.* London: HMSO, 1990.

7. OTHER EVENTS OF INTEREST IN 1990

(a) Primary health care

(i) Effects of the new contract

Improving the range and quality of services to patients has been the central theme for general medical services since the mid-1980s. However, the new contract for general practitioners (GPs), which became effective on 1 April 1990, was the first major revision of the contractual framework of the family doctor service for over 20 years. For the first time, health promotion and disease prevention are a formal part of the GP's contract with the National Health Service (NHS). Since it came into force the contract has influenced the pattern of primary health care significantly. In the first nine months under the new arrangements 461,000 separate health promotion clinics were held.

It is already possible to see other positive results of the changes brought about by the new contract. They include:

Cervical cytology and immunisation uptake

Table 7.1 shows the percentage of GPs who were achieving target payments for childhood immunisation and cervical cancer screening at the start of the new contract in April 1990. A GP qualifies for the higher target payment for immunisation if 90% of the children of the appropriate age registered with the practice are immunised, and the lower payment for immunising 70% of those children. The comparable targets for cervical cancer screening of eligible women are 80% and 50%.

The new contract has assisted in increasing the uptake of cervical smears in the vulnerable population. Because of the natural history of the disease, several years will elapse before reduction in mortality from cancer of the cervix—the true outcome measurement—can be demonstrated.

Table 7.1: *General practitioners receiving target payments for immunisation and cervical cytology, April 1990*

	GPs receiving target payment		
	Higher %	Lower %	Total %
Childhood immunisation	58	24	82
Pre-school booster	50	25	75
Cervical screening	55	33	88

Similarly, by November 1990 there had been an increase in the uptake of childhood immunisation, continuing the previous upward trend. The uptake of diphtheria, tetanus and polio vaccine was 90%, of pertussis vaccine 83%, and of measles vaccine 88%. The comparable figures for 1989 were 86%, 75% and 80% respectively.

Minor surgery

68% of GPs were admitted to the minor surgery list by their Family Health Services Authority (FHSA), qualifying them for payment for undertaking a specific range of treatments. In the first nine months of the new contract GPs held 83,000 minor surgery sessions during which they undertook almost half a million procedures. Prior to the new contract, the majority of these would have been undertaken in hospital outpatient departments, with the inconvenience to patients of waiting lists and greater distances to travel.

(ii) Computerisation in general practice

During 1990, there was a rapid increase of computerisation in general practice, aided by an additional allocation of £24 million to allow payments to be made directly to GPs buying systems. A survey in April showed that almost 60% of practices were using a computer, representing at least 59.5% of all GPs in England. The percentage of computerised practices increases with practice size, from 23% of single-handed practices to 96% of partnerships of six or more. GPs are using their systems for an increasing number of purposes, including the recording of clinical data and medicines prescribed during consultations, and for medical audit. They have also been using them to fulfil the 1990 contract, eg for call and recall programmes for health promotion and disease prevention, production of annual reports on practice activity, and assessment of whether targets have been reached for childhood immunisation and cervical cytology. Computerisation is a complex issue and guidance was issued by the Department of Health (DH) to all GPs[1]. Many FHSAs have appointed facilitators to help GPs computerise as effectively as possible.

(iii) Audit in the family health services

In June 1990 DH issued a Health Circular[2] which recommended that professionally led local groups (Medical Audit Advisory Groups (MAAGs)) should be established by FHSAs to encourage medical audit in general practice. Pilot projects started in 1989 had shown that, in order to have a greater influence, audit should make use of local resources and recognise local needs. During 1990, £11 million was provided for audit within FHSAs and nationwide projects were supported through the Royal College of General Practitioners (RCGP) and the General Medical Services Committee. FHSAs adopted many approaches, including the employment of facilitators, small team visiting, workshops, and other initiatives. Medical audit in primary care is developing a momentum of its own as GPs recognise its value to them and their patients.

(iv) Postgraduate education

Doctors have always been responsible for their own continuing postgraduate education and, in order to provide encouragement, the Government introduced the Postgraduate Education Allowance (PGEA) in the new contract. Previously only 45% of GPs regularly attended formal courses to keep up-to-date. Now, when a doctor has attended sufficient PGEA-approved educational activities, geared towards providing a high standard of care for patients, he or she becomes eligible for a substantial extra allowance. The allowance includes an element for expenses (course fees, travel etc), and an incentive element. If attendance can be judged an appropriate criterion, PGEA has been a major success; over 80% of GPs have attended a locally accredited course. Postgraduate advisers in general practice are responsible for approving the quality of the courses, and ensuring that local educational needs are met.

Education about mental illness

Following the success of the conference on *Counselling in General Practice*, described in the Report for 1989[3], DH organised two further conferences to educate primary health care teams about mental illness. The first was entitled *The Prevention of Depression and Anxiety—the role of the practice team*, and was held in collaboration with the RCGP and MIND. The second was on *The Primary Care of Schizophrenia*, and was held in collaboration with the RCGP and Research and Development in Psychiatry.

(v) Practice staff

The new contract gave FHSAs discretion to approve reimbursement of a proportion of the cost of employing a range of health care professionals, such as counsellors, physiotherapists, chiropodists, practice managers and link workers. Their discretion extends to such matters as variations in pay and reimbursement of training costs. As a result, FHSAs and practitioners have greater scope for targeting support to meet local needs.

In 1990, the number of practice nurses alone increased by over 60%. This will help primary health care teams (PHCTs) to extend the range of services they provide and release GP time for activities which demand medical skills. A large number of new secretarial staff also joined PHCTs, whose development will permit the evolution of better systems to handle the long-recognised challenges of health promotion and continuing care.

Facilitators

Facilitators, both lay and medical, have been employed to support the PHCT in the development and provision of services. They have specific expertise which can be passed on to the PHCT, and the National Facilitator Development project supports their professional development and training. There are now 172 primary health care facilitators in the field of health promotion, most of whom have a background of primary health care nursing. They are widely distributed throughout the country, and cover a potential population of 41 million people.

Medical and nursing facilitators assisting in the development of palliative and terminal care in general practice have previously worked with such organisations as the Marie Curie Foundation and the Macmillan Trust, and are able to give technical advice, loan equipment, and help staff gain confidence in work they may have delegated or referred in the past. Another example of facilitation is the work of doctors with medical audit expertise to explore avenues of development, and to support the setting up of audit schemes and the establishment of audit protocols.

References

1   Department of Health. *GP computing: information for GPs on Practice Computer Systems*. London: HMSO, 1990.

2   Department of Health. *Health service developments—Working for Patients: medical audit in the Family Practitioner Services*. London: Department of Health, 1990. (Circulars: HC(FP)(90)8; HC(90)15).

3   Department of Health. *On the State of the Public Health: the annual report of the Chief Medical Officer of the Department of Health for the year 1989*. London: HMSO, 1990; 130.

(b) Hospital services

(i) Accident and emergency and trauma services

Trauma centre evaluation

Following consultation on the Royal College of Surgeons (RCS) Report on *The Management of Patients with Major Injuries*[1], it was decided to establish a trauma centre evaluation project in England to help determine whether Regional Trauma Centres should be encouraged. Regions which had plans to include a trauma centre as part of their accident and emergency provision were invited to bid for additional funding.

Criteria for a pilot trauma centre were set with the help of an Advisory Group. These included a catchment population of around 2 million people, the availability of the essential specialties on site, a resident 24 hours-a-day consultant-led trauma team, resources already available to the unit, and a management commitment to the project. There were 13 applications. The Advisory Group selected the North Staffordshire Royal Infirmary, Stoke-on-Trent, as the pilot centre. Hull Royal Infirmary and the Royal Preston Hospital were chosen as comparators. Professor Brian Williams of Sheffield University will be evaluating the trauma care systems in each of these areas, beginning in April 1991.

Quality initiatives in accident and emergency

As part of an initiative to raise quality standards in hospitals and improve services to the public, DH agreed to provide £800,000 to support four demonstration projects in Accident and Emergency Departments in 1990/91. Regions were invited to submit bids and 33 applications were received. The Departments selected were those at the Hull Royal Infirmary, the Royal Preston Hospital, Peterborough District Hospital and Southend District Hospital. These projects include: improvements to the environment, particularly reception, waiting and treatment areas; reduction of waiting times; appointment of 'triage' nurses and nurse practitioners; and information for patients and improved customer relations.

(ii) Emergency planning in the National Health Service

In October 1990, DH published Health Circular HC(90)25[2] and guidance consolidating and updating earlier guidance on planning health service arrangements for dealing with major incidents. It replaced Health Circular HC(77)1. There had been a considerable demand for updated guidance in view of recent major incidents in this country. The new guidance was prepared jointly with representatives of health authorities and the ambulance services, and in consultation with professional and health service organisations.

The purpose of emergency planning is to ensure that health care services are prepared for an effective response to any major incident. The guidance indicates the need for an 'All Hazards' approach to planning which includes the identification and application of principles common to a spectrum of hazards. There is also a need to set out details for dealing with special risks in each area, such as motorways, airports, chemical plants and venues for sporting and other public events. Health authorities are required to ensure that there are comprehensive plans for dealing with major incidents in accordance with the revised guidance. From April 1991, all major incident plans will have to be secured by contractual arrangements, and take into account cross boundary arrangements and training.

(iii) Training of ambulance staff

If the number of people dying from heart attacks or severe accidental injury before reaching hospital is to be reduced, there is a need to improve pre-hospital care. Measures to achieve this include the further training of qualified ambulance staff and a substantial increase in the number of fully trained paramedics.

An additional £3.8 million was provided in July 1990 to allow all emergency ambulances to be equipped with a defibrillator. Deliveries should be complete by April 1991. By the end of 1991 all qualified ambulance staff should be trained in cardiopulmonary resuscitation and in the use of a defibrillator. Over the next 5-6 years, 60% of qualified ambulance staff should be trained to paramedic standard to enable every emergency ambulance to be staffed by at least one fully trained paramedic.

The National Health Service Training Authority (NHSTA) has revised the training manual for ambulance paramedics in consultation with the Joint Medical Colleges Ambulance Services Liaison Committee; the manual will be available in the spring of 1991. DH is contributing £20,000 per year to the administrative costs of the Liaison Committee in recognition of the contribution it is making towards the development and improvement of the emergency ambulance service.

(iv) Day surgery and minimally invasive therapy

Day surgery

On 19 October 1990 the Audit Commission published its report on day surgery[3]. DH is in broad agreement with the findings and conclusions of this report, which recommended that some 20 procedures (those highlighted in the 1985 RCS report[4]) should be customarily undertaken by day surgery. The report is seen as a further valuable contribution to the debate on day surgery. It emphasised that the most cost-effective way of providing day surgery was in dedicated day units.

Although the proportion of operations carried out by day surgery has risen steadily—from 570,000 day cases in 1979 to over a million in 1989/90—the proportion of particular operations performed by day surgery varies widely between Districts, within Districts, and between hospitals. Following publication of the DH report *The Management and Utilisation of Operating Departments*[5] in December 1989 and consultation on it, the Management Executive recommended in July 1990 that health authorities should issue guidelines and set targets for day surgery. In deciding whether day surgery is appropriate for an individual patient, the clinical judgement of the responsible doctor must be paramount.

Day surgery is being encouraged for three main reasons:

- Medical advances make it possible to carry out certain procedures more quickly and easily, sometimes with minimally invasive techniques and using local or regional anaesthesia rather than a general anaesthetic.

- It is preferable for the patient to be able to return to his or her home and family rather than have to stay in hospital.

- Research studies have shown that it is more cost-effective than inpatient treatment.

Minimally invasive therapy

The last decade has seen both rapid advances in technology and an increasing interest on the part of clinicians to reduce patient trauma and morbidity in all areas of clinical activity. A characteristic of this new approach to patient care has been the use of the endoscope by surgeons to widen its application to include operations on organs such as the appendix and the gall-bladder, so that patients now have only the smallest of incisions and a less profound anaesthetic.

1990 saw the first anniversary of the founding of the Society of Minimally Invasive Therapy, formed to bring together all the specialties developing expertise in this area. It is not only surgeons who are involved; radiologists are developing 'interventional techniques' and gastro-enterologists are extending their skills as technology improves. However, new techniques have to be learned and there is a parallel interest in teaching and training. The RCS, in welcoming the advances in this field, set out criteria for the training and provision of endoscopic surgery in a statement on minimal access surgery published in 1990[6].

(v) Ionising Radiation (Protection of Persons Undergoing Medical Examination or Treatment) Regulations 1988

The Ionising Radiation (Protection of Persons Undergoing Medical Examination or Treatment) Regulations 1988[7], colloquially known as POPUMET, implement European Community Directive 84/466/Euratom. As the title indicates, the Regulations are concerned with the protection of patients when ionising radiation is being used, and they complement the Ionising Radiations Regulations 1985[8], which are concerned with protecting staff.

In essence, the Regulations require medical exposures involving the use of ionising radiation to conform to accepted diagnostic or therapeutic practice; radiation doses to be as low as reasonably practicable; those using ionising radiation to undergo training in radiation protection as well as training in the practical aspects of the techniques being used; records of the training of staff to be kept; an inventory of equipment to be maintained; and the advice of a medical physicist to be available.

The training of staff to comply with the Regulations has been a major undertaking. The need for training will continue as newly qualified staff undertake procedures such as the injection of radiopharmaceuticals, or junior doctors insert temporary pacing wires in the coronary care unit under fluoroscopic control, or use fluoroscopy for setting a fracture in the operating theatre.

The Regulations use the phrase 'clinically directing' and define clinically directing as "having clinical responsibility for the decision to effect a medical exposure". This clinical responsibility includes responsibility for ensuring that the radiographic technique selected results in a radiation dose to the patient that is as low as reasonably practicable. The person who requests a medical exposure may well not be clinically directing. In diagnostic radiology, the radiologist is likely to be clinically directing, unless another clinician, such as a cardiologist performing cardiac catheterisation, is undertaking fluoroscopy. In nuclear medicine, it is the holder of a certificate issued by Ministers authorising a clinician or dentist to administer radiopharmaceuticals to a patient (an ARSAC certificate) who is likely to be clinically directing; and in radiotherapy it is likely to be the radiotherapist/clinical oncologist.

The Regulations use the phrase 'physically directing' to refer to the person who actually effects the medical exposure. In diagnostic radiology this will usually be a radiographer, although, if fluoroscopy is being undertaken, it could be the person who clinically directs. In radiotherapy, the person physically directing will be a radiographer.

The Regulations are enforced as health and safety regulations under the Health and Safety at Work Act 1974[9], and a breach of the Regulations is a criminal offence. The Health and Safety Executive is enforcing most of the Regulations, although Regulation 4 is being enforced by Inspectors appointed by the Secretary of State for Health. Regulation 4 is concerned with medical exposures being conducted in accordance with accepted diagnostic or therapeutic practice, and with ensuring that procedures are selected to ensure a dose of ionising radiation to the patient as low as reasonably practicable in order to achieve the required diagnostic or therapeutic purpose.

Incidents alleging possible infringement of this Regulation are being reported to the Inspectorate at a rate of more than one a month. Each is time-consuming, both for the Inspectorate and for the staff concerned with the incident. A number of difficult issues have come to light, including the question of who is clinically directing a mammography screening. Based on advice from the Royal College of Radiologists, this is the person who interprets the mammogram unless there is a written statement to the effect that some other person is clinically directing. Another issue has been the concept of 'accepted clinical practice'. Although there is much guidance available on what constitutes good practice, the question is whether it is possible to define behaviour which deviates so far as to constitute unacceptable practice. For example, in the current state of knowledge, is mammographic screening of asymptomatic women under the age of 50 years (outside a research protocol) or pre-employment chest radiography acceptable? Another example is whether it is possible to define acceptable radiation doses for different diagnostic and therapeutic procedures.

Whilst the record of safety for the use of ionising radiation in diagnostic and therapeutic practice in this country can be regarded as satisfactory, there is room for improvement (eg the elimination of unnecessary X-rays and the reduction of doses)[10]. Implementation of the Regulations should result in better protection for the patient.

References

1 Royal College of Surgeons of England. Working Party on the Management of Patients with Major Injuries. *Report of the Working Party on the Mangement of Patients with Major Injuries*. London: Royal College of Surgeons of England, 1988. Chairman: Professor Miles Irving.

2 *Emergency Planning in the NHS: Health Services Arrangements for Dealing with Major Incidents*. London: Department of Health, 1990. (Health Circular: HC(90)25).

3 Audit Commission. *A short cut to better services. Day surgery in England and Wales*. London: HMSO, 1990.

4 Royal College of Surgeons of England. *Guidelines for day case surgery*. London: Royal College of Surgeons, 1985.

5 Department of Health. NHS Management Executive VFM Unit. *The management and utilisation of operating departments*. London: Department of Health, 1989.

6 Royal College of Surgeons of England. *Minimal access surgery*. London: Royal College of Surgeons, 1990.

7 *Ionising Radiation (Protection of persons undergoing medical examinations or treatment) Regulations 1988*. London: HMS0, 1988.

8 *Ionising Radiations Regulations 1985*. London: HMSO, 1985.

9 *Health and Safety at Work Act 1974*. London HMSO, 1974.

10 *Patient dose reduction in diagnostic radiology*. Documents of the NRPB Volume 1 No 3 1990.

(c) Mental health

(i) Care Programmes, Specific Grant, and central London homeless mentally ill initiative

The reports for 1988 and 1989[1,2] referred to the need to ensure continuity of care for people with severe long-term mental illness when they leave hospital and are cared for in the community. Three recent developments should help ensure continuity of services, and improve the provision of health and social care to those mentally ill people who have fallen out of care into destitution and homelessness.

Care Programmes

Since 1988 it has been a service objective for the NHS to introduce by April 1991 'Care Programmes' to improve the delivery of services to people with severe mental illness. Care Programmes include an assessment of need, case management involving the appointment of a key worker, systematic review and appropriate follow-up. This approach is likely to be particularly beneficial to those people suffering from the more severe and chronic forms of mental illness. Guidance on the Care Programme approach has now appeared in the

171

form of a joint circular to health authorities and local authorities identifying the key components of the approach[3], and a companion set of published articles describing how each of these components can be put into effect in a working service[4,5,6].

Mental illness Specific Grant

Many seriously mentally ill people being cared for outside hospital need social care as well as health care. It is clear that local authorities have not so far been able to give services for the mentally ill a very high priority. At present, only some 3% of Social Services' expenditure is on services for mentally ill people. The National Health Service and Community Care Act 1990[7] provides for a Specific Grant to be paid to local authorities. It is to be used to encourage Social Services Departments to improve existing services, and develop new services to provide social care to the most severely mentally ill people. The Grant, to be introduced in 1991, will be payable only on the basis of plans jointly agreed by the local authority and the health authority, and so will be a powerful incentive to joint planning. It will support total expenditure of £30 million in the first year, the equivalent of at least 15% real growth in local authority resources devoted to mental illness[8].

Central London homeless mentally ill initiative

The Reports for 1987 and 1989[9,10] drew attention to the high prevalence of severe untreated mental illness evident among homeless people on the streets of central London. The better planning of hospital discharge and follow-up that will result from Care Programmes, and the greater availability of social care facilities resulting from the Specific Grants, should reduce the likelihood that in future people with mental illness, drug misuse or alcohol misuse will end up homeless and sleeping rough. A further initiative was announced on 12 July 1990 by Stephen Dorrell, Parliamentary Under Secretary of State for Health[11]. This will offer accommodation and psychiatric care to homeless mentally ill people in central London. The scheme is likely to cost more than £5 million over the first two years. It includes the provision of around 75 new specialist short-term hostel places with social support, and new community-based psychiatric teams in the three Thames Regions with central London Districts. The aim is first to contact, and then to help, homeless mentally ill people. The Housing Corporation will be looking to housing associations to provide up to 450 new housing places between 1991 and 1994, to which residents of the short-term hostels can progress. The community psychiatric teams are based on the successful model of the Lewisham and North Southwark Psychiatric Team for Single Homeless People[12]. Health and social services authorities in central London have been asked to collaborate with appropriate voluntary organisations to make a fuller assessment of the numbers of homeless mentally ill people, and to identify how their health and social care needs can be best met. The initiative will be evaluated, and the results should provide useful information for other parts of the country.

The Royal College of Psychiatrists has now published a Report of the *Working Conference on Homelessness,* organised jointly with DH in 1989. It makes a number of recommendations to improve the care provided by medical and other services to homeless people[13].

(ii) Suicide and avoidable mortality in young adults

While there has been a general downward trend over recent decades for suicide rates in both sexes over the complete age range, in young men the suicide rate is rising[14,15] (see Figure 7.1). These trends were described in the Report for 1989[16]. The United Kingdom (UK) is not unique in this respect as there is a similar trend in the USA and the rest of Europe[17,18,19].

Factors affecting the suicide rate

Researchers have looked for factors which increase or reduce the risk of individuals committing suicide, and factors that influence suicide rates for groups of people or populations. These approaches are complementary, and there appear to be many factors associated with suicide; they may operate in addition or in multiplication.

Key variables include mental disorder[20], alcohol and drug misuse[21], the percentage of the population aged over 65 years[22], employment and unemployment[17], imprisonment[23], migration[24,25], marital breakdown, AIDS[26], post-traumatic stress disorders (including combat neuroses), and changes in the availability of different methods of suicide.

It is not yet known whether the current increase in the suicide rate in young men is a period effect or a cohort effect[27,28]. The distinction is important because, if it is a cohort effect, the increase seen now in this age-group would be expected to spread to older age-groups later on. On the other hand, if it is a period effect, the explanations would be found among changes that have affected people in this particular age range during the 1970s and 1980s. It will only become clearer as this generation gets older. An association between unemployment and suicide in young men has been suggested[29,30,31,32], but the precise causal relationship is not yet clear. However, while there was a fall in unemployment from 3 million to 1.6 million in the UK during the late 1980s, there was no corresponding dip in the suicide rate of young men.

Marital breakdown may have both an immediate effect on suicide rates, and a delayed effect following its harmful impact on the children of parents who divorced before the children reached adulthood[33,34,35]. It should be noted that there was a rapid rise in the divorce rate in the 1960s and the children born then are now young adults. Immigration is another factor which may operate both at the individual level, because of stress and lack of social support in the new community, and at the population level because of the lack of cohesiveness of a society[22,25,36,37,38]. While there are increasing reports of suicide in young men with AIDS[26,39], the rise in the suicide rate in young men long pre-dated the AIDS epidemic; it is clear that the epidemic may offer only a partial explanation for the years since 1984. There is no evidence to support the notion that fear of AIDS is a key variable. Motherhood does not protect against depression, but it does seem to protect young women from suicide. If the recent rise in suicide in young people is a cohort effect, the suicide rate of middle-aged women may rise in the next two decades, as their child rearing responsibilities come to an end. The effects of mental disorder and alcohol abuse are illustrated by the suicide rates in schizophrenics (10%)[40], people with affective psychosis (15%)[41], and

Figure 7.1: *Suicide rates, England and Wales, 1901-89*

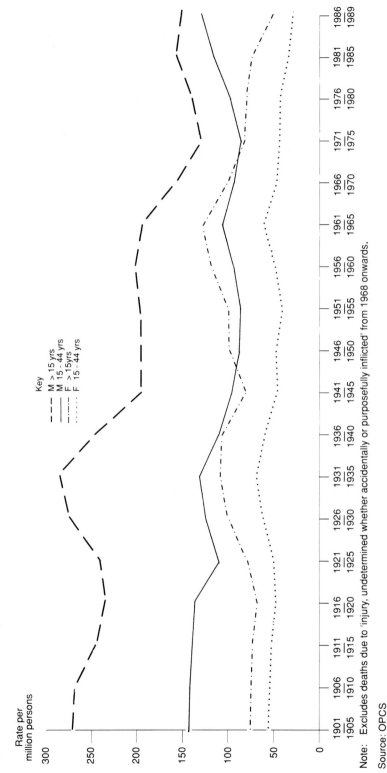

Note: Excludes deaths due to 'injury, undetermined whether accidentally or purposefully inflicted' from 1968 onwards.

Source: OPCS

174

alcoholics (15%)[21]. There is no evidence that serious mental disorder is increasing in the general population. However, alcohol and drug misuse are on the increase, and are often associated with marital breakdown and unemployment.

The availability of easy methods of suicide is known to be an important factor in influencing suicide rates, as exemplified by the fall in suicide rates in the early 1960s following the reduction of the proportion of carbon monoxide in coal gas[27]. In contrast, inhalation of car exhaust fumes has increased dramatically in recent years, and parallels the increased availability of the motor car, and the hatchback in particular[14], probably because it is easier to run a tube from the exhaust pipe into the car. While self-poisoning as a method of suicide has declined in recent years, in parallel with reduced prescriptions for barbiturates, suicide by hanging and other violent means is also rising, with no obvious explanation (see Figures 7.2 and 7.3).

Prison suicides

In 1990, as the result of his concern about the steady increase in the number of suicides amongst prisoners, the Home Secretary asked Her Majesty's Chief Inspector of Prisons, His Honour Judge Tumim, to carry out a review of suicide and self-harm in Prison Service Establishments. The Report[42] was published in December 1990.

It recorded an increase in the number of self-inflicted deaths from 29 in 1985 to 48 in 1989. Of the 48 deaths in 1989, 33 were confirmed as suicide by the Coroner's Court. The 1988 figure of 30 confirmed suicides amongst prisoners is compared with the total number of suicides in the UK in the same year. The incidence based on the daily prison population was about six times higher than the national average. The Report states that the majority of prisoners who committed suicide were not mentally disordered within the meaning of the Mental Health Act 1983. This reflects the findings of previous research. The implications for the NHS, the Special Hospitals Service Authority and local authorities arising from this Report, the Woolf Report into the Strangeways Prison disturbances, and the Efficiency Scrutiny of the Prison Medical Service[43] will be considered by the Review of Services for Mentally Disordered Offenders announced by the Parliamentary Under Secretary of State for Health in November 1990[44].

A joint Home Office and DH Steering Committee, chaired by the head of DH's Mental Health, Elderly and Disability Division, Dr John Reed, will examine the need for changes in the current level, pattern and operation of health and social services for mentally disordered offenders.

Avoidable mortality

Apart from suicide, there is also an avoidable mortality from other causes among those who have suffered from mental illness. Fox and Goldblatt have demonstrated the grossly elevated standard mortality ratios of people in the years following their discharge from mental hospitals, largely due to cardio-vascular disease, respiratory disease and malignancy[45]. In mental handicap, while deaths from status epilepticus and respiratory infections have decreased,

Figure 7.2: *Number of male suicides aged 15-44 years by method of suicide, England and Wales, 1950-89*

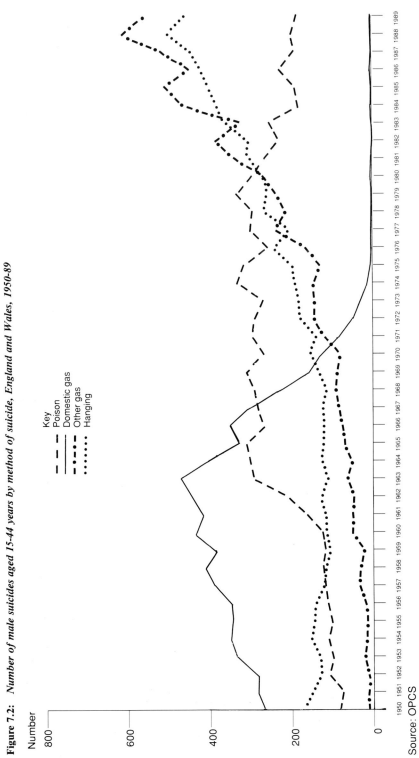

Source: OPCS

Figure 7.3: *Number of female suicides aged 15-44 years by method of suicide, England and Wales, 1950-89*

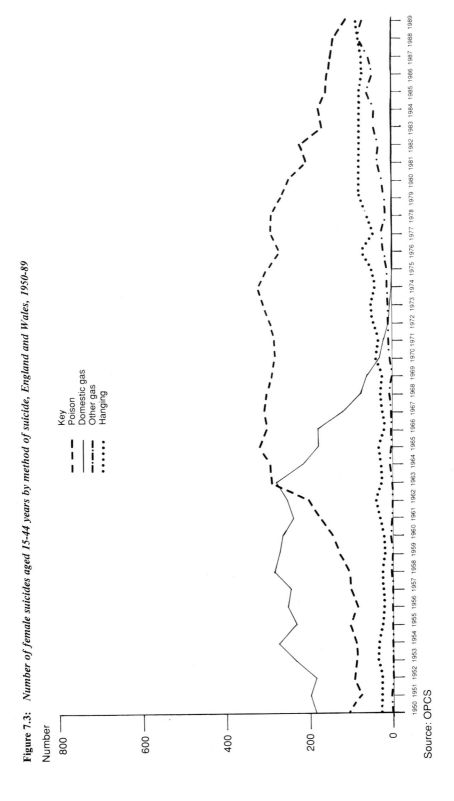

Source: OPCS

deaths due to carcinoma (particularly gastro-intestinal), myocardial infarction and cerebrovascular accident have increased[46].

References

1 Department of Health and Social Security. *On the State of the Public Health: the annual report of the Chief Medical Officer of the Department of Health and Social Security for the year 1987*. London: HMSO, 1988; 69-73.

2 Department of Health. *On the State of the Public Health: the annual report of the Chief Medical Officer of the Department of Health for the year 1988*. London: HMSO, 1989; 174-5.

3 Department of Health. *The care programme approach for people with a mental illness referred to the specialist psychiatric services*. London: Department of Health, 1990. (Circular: HC(90)23/LASSL(90)11).

4 Shepherd G. Case management. *Health Trends* 1990; **22**: 59-62.

5 Burns T. Community ward rounds. *Health Trends* 1990; **22**: 62-3.

6 Harborne G, Henderson A. Case registers. *Health Trends 1990;* **22**: 63-4.

7 *National Health Service and Community Care Act 1990*. London: HMSO, 1990.

8 Department of Health. *Specific grant for the development of social care services for people with a mental illness*. London: Department of Health, 1990. (Circulars: HC(90) 24; LAC(90)10).

9 Department of Health and Social Security. *On the State of the Public Health: the annual report of the Chief Medical Officer of the Department of Health and Social Security for the year 1987*. London: HMSO, 1988; 71-2.

10 Department of Health. *On the State of the Public Health: the annual report of the Chief Medical Officer of the Department of Health for the year 1989*. London: HMSO, 1990; 130.

11 Department of Health. *Stephen Dorrell announces new scheme to help homeless and mentally ill people in London*. London: Department of Health, 1990. (Press Release 90/352).

12 The psychiatric team for single homeless people. *Plugging the gaps: providing a service for homeless mentally ill people*. London: Lewisham and North Southwark Health Authority, 1990.

13 Royal College of Psychiatrists. *Mental Health and Homelessness*. London: Royal College of Psychiatrists, 1990. (Occasional Paper OP9).

14 Bulusu L, Alderson M. Suicides 1950. *Population Trends* 1984; **35**: 11-7.

15 Monk M. Epidemiology of suicide. *Epidemiol Rev* 1987; **9**: 51-70.

16 Department of Health. *On the State of the Public Health: the annual report of the Chief Medical Officer of the Department of Health for the year 1989*. London: HMSO, 1990; 2, 152.

17 Pritchard C. Suicide, gender and unemployment in the British Isles and EEC 1974-1985. *Soc Psychiatry Psychiatr Epidemiol* 1988; **23**: 85-9.

18 Klerman GL, ed. *Suicide and depression among adolescents and young adults*. Washington DC: American Psychiatric Press, 1986.

19 Solomon MI, Hellon CP. Suicide and age in Alberta, Canada 1951-1977. A cohort analysis. *Arch Gen Psychiatry* 1980; **37**: 511-3.

20 Barraclough B, Burch J, Nelson B et al. A hundred cases of suicides: clinical aspects. *Br J Psychiatry* 1974; **125**: 355-73.

21 Raj A, Linnoila M. Alcoholism and suicide. *Suicide Life Threat Behav* 1986; **16**: 244-73.

22 Trovato F. A time series analysis of international immigration and suicide mortality in Canada. *International Journal of The Society of Psychiatry* 1986; **32**: 38-46.

23 Dooley E. Prison suicide in England and Wales 1972-87. *Br J Psychiatry* 1990; **156**: 40-5.

24 Lester D. *Why people kill themselves: A summary of research findings on suicidal behaviour*. Springfield, Illinois: Thomas, 1983.

25 Kushner HI. Immigrant suicide in the United States: Toward a psycho-social history. *Journal of Social History* 1984; **18**: 3-24.

26 Marzuk PM, Tierney H, Tardiff K et al. Increased risk of suicide in persons with AIDS. *JAMA* 1988; **159**: 1333-7.

27 Murphy E, Lindesay J, Grundy E. 60 years of suicide in England and Wales. *Arch Gen Psychiatry* 1986; **43**: 969-76.

28 Wetzel RD, Reich T, Murphy GE, Province M, Miller JP. The changing relationship between age and suicide rates: cohort effect, period effect or both? *Psychiatric Dev* 1987; **3**: 179-218.

29 Crombie IK. Trends in suicide and unemployment in Scotland 1976-1986. *Br Med J* 1989; **298**: 782-4.

30 Platt S. Unemployment and suicidal behaviour: A review of the literature. *Soc Sci Med* 1984; **2**: 93-115.

31 Day LH. Death from non-war violence: an international comparison. *Soc Sci Med* 1984; **2**: 917-27.

32 Horwitz AV. The economy and social pathology. *Annual Review of Sociology* 1984; **10**: 95-119.

33 Stack S. The effects of marital dissolution on suicide. *Journal of Marriage and the Family* 1980; **42**: 83-92.

34 Wassoma IM. A longitudinal analysis of the linkage between suicide, unemployment and marital dissolution. *Journal of Marriage and the Family* 1984; **46**: 855-9.

35 Jacobson GF, Portuges SH. Relation of marital separation and divorce to suicide: a report. *Suicide Life Threat Behav* 1978; **8**: 217-24.

36 Lester D. Suicide risk by birth cohort. *Suicide Life Threat Behav* 1984; **14**: 132-6.

37 Brahimi M. La mortalité des étrangers en France. *Populations* 1980; **35**: 603-22.

38 Whitlock FA. Migration and suicide. *Med J Aust* 1971; **2**: 840-8.

39 McCormick A. Trends in mortality statistics in England and Wales with particular reference to AIDS from 1984 to April 1987. *Br Med J* 1988; **296**: 1289-92.

40 Hawton K. Assessment of suicide risk. *Br J Psychiatry* 1987; **150**: 145-53.

41 Miles CP. Conditions predisposing to suicide: a review. *J Nerv Ment Dis* 1977; **164**: 231-46.

42 Home Office. *Report of a review by Her Majesty's Chief Inspector of Prisons for England and Wales of Suicide and Self Harm in prison service establishments in England and Wales.* London: HMSO, 1990.

43 Home Office. *Report of an efficiency scrutiny of the Prison Medical Service.* London: Home Office, 1990.

44 Department of Health. *Stephen Dorrell announces review of services for mentally disordered offenders.* London: Department of Health, 1990. (Press Release 90/581).

45 Fox AJ, Goldblatt PO. *Longitudinal study—Sociodemographic Mortality Differential LS No 1, 1971-1975.* London: HMSO, 1982.

46 Jancar J. Consequences of longer life for the mentally handicapped. *Geriatric medicine* 1988; **18**: 81-7.

(d) Disability and rehabilitation

Since 1986 there have been significant developments in the fields of disability and rehabilitation. Of particular note have been the publication of the Office of Population Censuses and Surveys (OPCS) surveys of disability; the publication of two reports by the Royal College of Physicians (RCP); and the creation of the Disablement Services Authority (DSA).

The OPCS surveys of disability in Great Britain were carried out between 1985 and 1988 and were published as a series of six reports between 1988 and 1989[1]. The reports provided information about the number of disabled people in Great Britain and their circumstances. The first report considered the prevalence of disability among adults[2] and estimated there were over 6 million people (14.2%) in the adult population with one or more significant disabilities. The surveys demonstrated how the overall rate of disability increases with age and that 70% of disabled adults were over 60 years-of-age; they also provided estimates of the prevalence of disability by type of disability (see Figure 7.4).

The publication in 1986 of the RCP report on *Physical Disability in 1986 and Beyond*[3] was a significant landmark, and was followed by the publication, in November 1990, of the RCP report *Health Services for Adults with Physical Disabilities*[4]. The latter was a descriptive study of NHS facilities and services provided for physically disabled adults in 183 English and 9 Welsh Districts.

Much of the information was not previously available. The OPCS surveys and the RCP reports, along with information from a variety of other sources[5,6,7,8,9,10,11], provide health authorities with valuable information concerning the planning and purchasing of rehabilitation services.

In 1990, rehabilitation medicine was recognised as a specialty by DH and the RCP. The Joint Planning Advisory Committee allocated an additional 15 senior registrar posts to rehabilitation medicine, bringing the total to 24 in all. However, there are only two professorial units of rehabilitation medicine in England—at Southampton and Leeds. Future progress in training, research and setting standards will crucially depend on the specialty developing further in these and other academic centres, so that a critical mass of workers from different professions provides the basis for future expansion.

Figure 7.4: *Estimates of prevalence of disability among adults by type of disability, Great Britain*

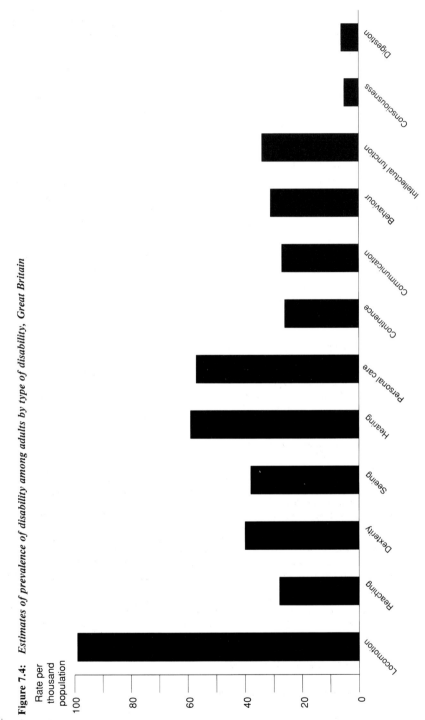

Source: OPCS

180

The DSA was established in 1987, following publication of the McColl report[12], to take over the Artificial Limb and Appliance Service previously administered by the Department of Health and Social Security, and to integrate this service into the NHS in 1991. The Authority is strongly committed to the development of a comprehensive rehabilitation service, and believes that the integration of disablement services within the NHS offers an opportunity for the development of rehabilitation. The Chief Medical Officer highlighted the importance of rehabilitation in an integrated health care service when he addressed, in October 1990, a conference on the *National Concept of Rehabilitation Medicine*, jointly arranged by the RCP and the DSA.

April 1990 saw the introduction of a major revision of Form BD8 for the certification of blind and partially sighted people. The new form and new procedures were introduced following recommendations in the Working Group report *Co-ordinating Services for Visually Handicapped People*[13], published in 1989. The epidemiological section of the form was revised to allow collection of better information on the causes of blindness and partial sight. The collection, analysis and publication of statistical data on the causes of blindness and partial sight was transferred to OPCS at the same time. The new form is designed to improve service delivery at local authority level, inter-agency collaboration and statistical information, and should be a significant step forward in the provision of services to visually handicapped people.

References

1   Martin J, Meltzer H, Elliot D. *OPCS surveys of disability in Great Britain*. London: HMSO, 1988-1989. Six reports.

2   Martin J, Meltzer H, Elliot D. *The prevalence of disability among adults. OPCS surveys of disability in Great Britain: Report 1*. London: HMSO, 1988.

3   Royal College of Physicians. *Physical disability in 1986 and beyond. A report of the Royal College of Physicians*. London: Royal College of Physicians, 1986.

4   Edwards FC, Warren MD. *Health services for adults with physical disabilities. A survey of district health authorities 1988/89*. London: Royal College of Physicians, 1990.

5   Department of Health. *The development of services for people with physical or sensory disabilities*. London: Department of Health, 1988. (Health Notice: HN (88)26).

6   Medical Disability Society. *The management of traumatic brain injury. A working party report of the Medical Disability Society*. London: The Development Trust for Young Disabled, 1988.

7   Royal College of Physicians. *Stroke. Towards better management. A report of the Royal College of Physicians*. London: Royal College of Physicians, 1989.

8   Wade DT, Langton Hewer R. Epidemiology of some neurological diseases with special reference to the workload on the NHS. *Int Rehabil Med* 1989; **8**: 129-37.

9   Royal College of Physicians. *The young disabled adult. The use of residential homes and hospital units for the age group 16-64. A report of the Royal College of Physicians*. London: Royal College of Physicians, 1986.

10 Shorvon SD. Medical assessment and treatment of chronic epilepsy. *Br Med J* 1991; **302**: 363-6.

11 Davis AC. The prevalence of hearing impairment and reported hearing disability among adults in Great Britain. *Int J Epidemiol* 1989; **18**: 911-7.

12 Department of Health and Social Security. *Review of artificial limb and appliance centre services. The report of an independent working party under the chairmanship of Professor Ian McColl*. London: DHSS, 1986.

13 *Co-ordinating services for visually handicapped peiople: report to the Minister for the Disabled*. London: HMSO, 1989.

(e) Maternity and child health services

(i) Human Fertilisation and Embryology Act 1990

The Human Fertilisation and Embryology (HF and E) Bill, to which reference was made in the Report for 1989[1], completed its passage through Parliament and was enacted on 1 November 1990[2]. The provisions for the control of the creation and use of human embryos outside the body, and the donation and storage of gametes and embryos, are in line with the recommendations of the report of the Committee of Inquiry chaired by Dame Mary (now Baroness) Warnock, published in 1984[3]. Whether research on human embryos should be permitted was the subject of long debates and a free vote in each of the Houses of Parliament. There were substantial majorities in favour of its continuation under licence from a Statutory Authority to be established under the Act.

The underlying matters with which the Act is concerned are those of status, ie status of the embryo in vitro and status of individuals born following the use of donated gametes. Clinical practice in this context is to be controlled by the Statutory Licensing Authority for HF and E, rather than by the legislation itself. Thus, although such control is a new departure, not found in any other field of clinical practice, a degree of flexibility is maintained because the control will be exerted largely by means of a Code of Practice to be issued by the Licensing Authority. The Code will serve as guidance for doctors and other professionals working in licensed clinical services and they will be expected to heed it.

The HF and E Authority was appointed in shadow form in July 1990, under the chairmanship of Professor Colin Campbell, a layman and Vice-Chancellor of the University of Nottingham. Its membership includes not only doctors and embryologists, but also individuals whose principal interests are in ethics and social science. The Authority immediately began preparing its Code of Practice, which must be approved by the Secretary of State and laid before Parliament.

One procedure covered by the Act is the biopsy of embryos. This has been successfully achieved, along with the development of a reliable method of determining their sex by examining the genetic structure[4]. Furthermore, at the Hammersmith Hospital, where this work was carried out, some of the biopsied embryos, known to be free of particular gene defects because they were female, have been transferred to women and live births have resulted. As more progess is made, it will be necessary to consider the contribution in vitro fertilisation may offer towards giving women the choice of avoiding the birth of children with serious handicaps. Until now its priority has been considered only in relation to its value as a means of alleviating some forms of infertility.

During the Bill's passage through the House of Commons, Members of Parliament sought to amend the Abortion Act 1967[5]. As a result the HF and E Act includes a section amending the 1967 Act in several respects. The most notable are the introduction of a new 24-week gestational time limit for most abortions, and of a new ground for abortion—grave permanent injury to the physical or mental health of the pregnant woman. This new ground, and the existing ground of substantial risk that, if the child were born, it would suffer from such physical or mental abnormalities as to be seriously handicapped, are without time limit. The section also makes clear that selective termination of pregnancy (termination of one or more, but not all, fetuses of a multiple pregnancy) may be performed if the requirements of the Abortion Act are fulfilled.

(ii) Confidential Enquiry into Stillbirths and Deaths in Infancy

A Working Group was set up by the Chief Medical Officer in September 1989

"to consider and report on the issues raised by the proposal to introduce confidential enquiry into stillbirths and deaths in infancy, and to make recommendations".

Establishment of the Working Group fulfilled a commitment in the Government Reply to the First Report from the Social Services Committee, Session 1988/89, on Perinatal, Neonatal and Infant Mortality[6], in response to persisting concerns about the marked geographical and socio-economic variations in infant mortality rates, the high prevalence of babies of low birthweight, and deaths attributed to sudden infant death syndrome[7].

The overall aim of confidential enquiry is to improve understanding of the factors relating to the death being investigated, and of ways in which the risks of death might be diminished, particularly with regard to avoidable factors. It might, therefore, investigate known risk factors; whether care known to reduce the risks in individual cases had actually been provided, and was appropriate and accessible; or whether there were elements of care and service provision whose quality had fallen below accepted standards. Confidential enquiry is particularly concerned with quality assurance. It encompasses clinical audit and the scrutiny of other factors which influence the overall quality of care.

A cardinal feature is an assessment of the presence of avoidable factors in the circumstances of a death. This is not to suggest that death could have been prevented in all cases in which avoidable factors are considered to have been present. However, the presence of an avoidable factor is an indication that the risk of death could have been at least reduced. Except when the avoidable factor was the result of unforeseen circumstances, or an inescapable series of events, its presence implies that there was some aspect of care which fell short of what should be expected, and which might have contributed to the fatal outcome[8,9].

Detailed enquiry into individual deaths, with a view to assessing antecedent factors, the circumstances of death, and related provision and delivery of care, requires access to sensitive information. This includes personal health information, and information which might reflect the judgements and actions of health professionals and of service managers. It is essential that the confidentiality of such information is maintained; the success of an enquiry depends on the strict observance of assurances that confidentiality will be protected, on the arrangements to limit access to confidential documents, and on the demonstration that those arrangements are sound. The findings of confidential enquiry are expected to guide clinical practice, including teaching and training; health authorities and service providers in assessing and meeting the needs of populations; and the Government in making policy.

The Working Group's report and recommendations have been considered by Ministers, and it is hoped that consultation with representatives of the professional bodies and NHS management will take place early in the summer of 1991.

(iii) Brain damaged babies

The steady reduction in perinatal mortality has encouraged the belief that the same beneficial influences—in particular the skills of midwives and obstetricians, and of paediatricians in the care of the newborn—should also have led to a reduction in the prevalence of child disability. Certain causes of disability, such as congenital rubella and Rhesus haemolytic disease, are now almost things of the past, but the trend for cerebral palsy has been disappointing. Figure 7.5, which is taken from a study in the Mersey Region[10], shows how falling stillbirth and perinatal mortality rates have not been matched by a corresponding fall in the prevalence of cerebral palsy. In fact, in infants of low birthweight and very low birthweight, the prevalence has risen.

Cerebral palsy

Surveys have shown that about 1 in 400 children have cerebral palsy, which is a non-progressive disability usually manifested as impaired control of movement and posture[11]. However, it may also be associated with delayed development, defective vision and hearing, difficulties with speech, or epilepsy. Fortunately many of the affected children have minimal disability and are able to function well in society; 50% have normal intelligence[12]. Tragically, some have profound multiple physical disabilities, often with severe mental retardation: these children require lifelong care.

In most instances the cause is not known. Uncommon causes include unavoidable disasters in pregnancy; certain childhood infections; and rare disorders of metabolism and other genetic conditions. But these explain only a small minority of cases. In some babies cerebral palsy is associated with retarded

Figure 7.5: *Stillbirth, perinatal mortality and cerebral palsy rates, Mersey Region, 1974-84*

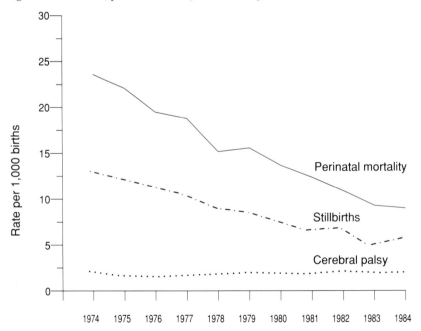

intra-uterine growth, and in others with congenital malformations, suggesting that abnormal development early in pregnancy was the cause in these infants. It is not known whether cerebral palsy has a similar cause in other infants, most of whom are of normal birthweight and appear to have had an uneventful pre-natal life and birth.

Following the misinterpretation of a paper published by William Little in 1862[13], the view became established that in the great majority of cases there is a causal relationship between perinatal events, especially birth asphyxia, and subsequent neurological impairment in the child. This view has persisted to the present time[14]. Moreover, it is often alleged that such damage is the result of obstetric negligence and that it was avoidable[15].

Most of these early studies were flawed by bias, small samples and inadequate control for confounding factors (particularly the strong relationship between low birthweight or low gestational age and adverse perinatal events, notably asphyxia, and cerebral palsy). In recent years a number of well-conducted studies have led to critical reappraisals of the evidence. They indicate that there is no evidence to support the belief that the quality of care during labour and delivery commonly influences the risk of cerebral palsy, nor that there is a strong relationship between cerebral palsy and putative indicators of birth asphyxia, whether preventable or not[16].

Unfortunately the persistence of earlier false beliefs has unwanted conse-quences. When a child is found to have cerebral palsy it is commonly supposed to be the result of obstetric mismanagement. It is not surprising therefore that litigation often follows. The trend in litigation, and the burden of its threat, are familiar[17]. They have evoked a number of concerns, among them the possibility that young doctors will be less inclined to specialise in obstetrics, with serious consequences for maternity services[15]. It is to be hoped that a wider apprecia-tion of the recent evidence concerning the causes of cerebral palsy should lead to a reversal of the litigious trend. It should also stimulate a renewed effort to seek the causes of this disability in pregnancy rather than during delivery.

These issues were discussed by the Chief Medical Officer in the 1990 William Power Memorial Lecture to the Royal College of Midwives.

(iv) Integration of child health services

Integration of child health services has long been recognised as essential to the delivery of high quality medical services for children. The Court Report[18] recommended in 1976 that there should be a family centred integrated child health service.

Historically, the organisation of secondary care for children has been divided between the hospital service and the community health service. The hospital service has concentrated on diagnosis and treatment, whilst preventive care and health surveillance have been provided largely by staff working in a separate community child health service. What is required is an extensive range of services for children of all ages—an integrated service that promotes child health through disease prevention, early detection of abnormality, and diag-nosis and treatment of acute illness. It must include the care of children in need, including children with disabilities, support of families, and the protection of children from abuse.

Artificial separation of services is not helpful. An integrated child health service should facilitate the provision of a comprehensive service and be consultant led. There needs to be an effective management structure to ensure the efficient deployment of staff and resources across the full range of services, including co-ordination of the contributions made by both health service professionals and staff of other agencies concerned with the health and welfare of children, eg Social Services Departments and Local Education Authorities.

During 1990, DH discussed with the British Paediatric Association (BPA) and other interested bodies the implications of the NHS reforms for child health services. In August 1989 the former Secretary of State for Health, Kenneth Clarke, in a letter to Professor Dame June Lloyd, then President of the BPA, had emphasised the Government's continuing commitment to an integrated hospital and community health service as the basis for good quality child health care. A joint working party of representatives of DH, the British Medical Association and the Conference of Medical Royal Colleges and Faculties will begin considering early in 1991 how a unified career structure for hospital and community health doctors working in child health may be created.

Under the new contracting arrangements, District Health Authorities (DHAs) are expected to specify that children and their families should receive integrated health care. It will be for provider units to decide on the organisational and management arrangements which will best enable them to deliver the standard of service required by the DHA. The quality of service received is all important and, while the inclusion of hospital and community children's services in a single management unit offers a proven organisational model, it is not the only option for the integration of child health services at the point of delivery. Some providers have chosen to create a community health management unit, including community child health medical staff and health visitors, separate from the hospital services. However, the hospital paediatricians and com-munity medical staff remain within the same clinical directorate. They provide for continuity of care for children and their families across primary and secondary services through agreement of common clinical policies which take account of the role of GPs.

It is essential that sound procedures for liaison and co-ordination are estab-lished, not only between staff working with children in hospital and community units (whether directly managed or within NHS Trusts), but also with GPs, whose involvement in child health surveillance is increasing. The reliability of these communication arrangements will be a key factor in the DHA's monitor-ing of the child health services it purchases.

(v) The Children Act 1989

The Children Act 1989[19] received Royal Assent on 16 November 1989 and will be implemented on 14 October 1991. It is the most comprehensive piece of legislation about children ever enacted, and represents a milestone in their care, upbringing and protection. The Act draws together and simplifies existing legislation to produce a practical and consistent code, integrating the law relating to private individuals with the responsibilities of public authorities towards children. In doing so, the Act strikes a new balance between family autonomy and the protection of children. For the first time there is a comprehensive and fully integrated scheme of private and public child law which recognises the welfare of the child as paramount, whilst ensuring fairness for parents and stressing family upbringing.

Much emphasis is laid on partnership between parents and local authorities, with children and parents participating in decision making about themselves. There is a range of new Court Orders designed to emphasise the continuing responsibility of both parents in the child's upbringing, combined with a more flexible system for hearing cases and inviting parental participation in the courts. *Working Together*[20], the guide to interagency co-operation in child protection, will be revised to reflect the changes brought about by the Act.

All NHS staff involved in the care of children need to be fully aware of the clear responsibilities that are laid down. DH recognises the key role the NHS will play in the successful implementation of the Act, especially in the planning and review of local authorities' arrangements for looking after individual children (including those with disabilities) and child protection. Initial awareness of the Act has been raised by the Department's publication *An Introduction to the Children Act*[21], which is aimed at providing a general understanding of the Act and its underlying principles. Draft Regulations and guidance documents relating to particular aspects of the Act have been disseminated widely for consultation, following which a series of Departmental guidance books, supported by individually commissioned good practice guidelines, will be published. In addition DH funded the National Children's Bureau to stage a series of Regional seminars for NHS senior managers and health professionals; the purpose was to raise awareness further and to emphasise the importance of collaboration between the health authorities and local authorities. They identified a number of local training needs.

Good training materials are vital to successful implementation of the Act. Some of the general training materials produced for local authorities can also be used by health authorities, but training materials and programmes are also needed specifically for health professionals working with children. To meet this need the Department has commissioned training material for NHS staff, together with a guide dealing with the Act's main provisions and its specific implications for health professionals.

References

1   Department of Health. *On the State of the Public Health: the annual report of the Chief Medical Officer of the Department of Health for the year 1989*. London: HMSO, 1990; 131.

2   *Human Fertilisation and Embryology Act 1990*. London: HMSO, 1990.

3   Committee of Enquiry into Human Fertilization and Embryology. *Report*. London: HMSO, 1984. (Cm. 9314). Chairman: Dame Mary Warnock.

4   Handyside AH et al. Biopsy of human preimplantation embryos and sexing by DNA amplification. *Lancet* 1989; **i**: 347-9.

5   *Abortion Act 1967*. London: HMSO, 1967.

6   Department of Health. *Perinatal, neonatal and infant mortality: Government reply to the First Report from the Social Services Committee, session 1988-89*. London: HMSO, 1989.

7   *Infant mortality in England: a report to the Chief Medical Officer by an expert working group*. London: Department of Health and Social Security, 1988.

8   Department of Health. *Report on confidential enquiries into maternal deaths in England and Wales 1982-84.* London: HMSO, 1989.

9   Brick N, Devlin HB, Lunn JN. *The report of a confidential enquiry into perioperative deaths.* London: Nuffield Provincial Hospitals Trust and King's Fund Trust, 1988. Chairman: MD Vickers.

10 Pharoah POD, Cooke T, Cooke RWI, Rosenbloom L. Birthweight specific trends in cerebral palsy. *Arch Dis Child* 1990; **65:** 602-6.

11 Pharoah POD. The epidemiology of cerebral palsy. *Seminars in Orthopaedics* 1989; **4:** 205-14.

12 *Oxford region register of early childhood impairments. Annual Report 1989.* Oxford: Oxford Region Child Development Project, 1989.

13 Little WJ. On the influence of abnormal parturition, difficult labours, premature birth and asphyxia neonatorum, on the mental and physical condition of the child, especially in relation to deformities. *Transactions of the Obstetric Society of London* 1861-62; **3:** 293-344.

14 Hey E. Fetal Hypoxia and Subsequent handicap: the problem of establishing a causal link. In: Chamberlain GVP, Orr CJB, Sharp F, eds. *Litigation Obstetrics and Gynaecology.* London: Royal College of Obstetricians and Gynaecologists, 1985.

15 Symonds EM. Obstetric nemesis. *Journal of the Medical Defence Union* 1989; **15:** 52-4.

16 Cerebral palsy, intrapartum care, and a shot in the foot. Editorial. *Lancet* 1989; **ii:** 1251-2.

17 Medical negligence: addressing the issues. *Proceedings of the Medical Protection Society Symposium, 13 December 1988.* London: The Medical Protection Society, 1989.

18 Department of Health and Social Security, Department of Education and Science and Welsh Office. *Fit for the future: report of Committee on Child Health Services.* London: HMSO, 1976. (Cm. 6684). Chairman: Professor SM Court.

19 *The Children Act 1989.* London: HMSO, 1989.

20 Department of Health and Social Security and Welsh Office. *Working Together: a guide to arrangements for inter-agency co-operation for the protection of children from abuse.* London: HMSO, 1988.

21 Department of Health. *An introduction to the Children Act 1989: a new framework for the care and upbringing of children.* London: HMSO, 1989.

(f) Medical manpower and education

(i) Junior doctors' hours

On 17 December 1990, the Ministerial Group on Junior Doctors' Hours, chaired by the Minister for Health, signed an agreement to reduce the hours worked by junior hospital doctors[1,2]. Under the agreement junior doctors will move towards a maximum average of 72 contracted hours per week. The short-term goal is a maximum average of 83 contracted hours per week. Taking into account time spent on-call, the number of hours actually worked should be considerably fewer. As workloads and staffing patterns vary so much between different hospitals, specialties and grades of doctor, the agreement sets out a package of mechanisms for change. Further guidance will be issued in the summer of 1991. This will enable those concerned at local level to solve the problems of both excessive total hours and over-long periods of continuous duty. Regional Task Forces are being established to propose solutions where local difficulties cannot easily be resolved. Considerable emphasis is being placed on the need to change working patterns. The measures being considered include full and partial shift working, greater use of cross-cover by juniors, more flexible deployment of medical staff, and making the optimum use of the skills of non-medical staff in the best interests of patient care.

To support the initiative, the Government is funding 200 new consultant and 50 new staff grade posts in England in 1991/92 as part of a rolling programme. The new posts will be carefully targeted to achieve the maximum impact on juniors' hours. They will help improve the quality of patient care, and are consistent with the ongoing programme to reform the hospital medical career structure. The agreement has the backing of the representatives of consultants and junior doctors, the medical Royal Colleges, the four UK Health

188

Departments and NHS management; all are represented on the Ministerial Group, which will continue to meet to ensure progress in the reduction of junior doctors' hours.

(ii) 'Achieving a Balance'

Achieving a Balance: Plan for Action[3], published in 1987, outlined a package of measures aimed to improve both patient care and the hospital medical staffing career structure. The basic principle underlying the package was the need to bring the number of doctors in the training grades more closely in line with future consultant opportunities. The package is being implemented over a 10-year period. The main measures include maintenance of existing rates of consultant expansion (an overall expansion of at least 2% per year, excluding any extra initiatives). A pump-priming scheme allocated 100 consultant posts during the period 1987-89, targeted at particular specialties. The Report also recommended the introduction of a new non-consultant career grade of hospital doctor, the 'staff grade'. The staff grade posts are being phased in gradually over a 10-year period until a ceiling of 10% of the number of consultants in post has been reached.

In 1990, considerable progress was made in implementing *Achieving a Balance*. The consultant grade expanded by 3% during 1989/90, comparing favourably with the expansion of 2.8% in 1988/89; it was well in excess of 2%, even when account is taken of the pump-priming posts and the 100 new consultant posts announced in the White Paper *Working for Patients*[4]. The rate of uptake for the staff grade during its first year of implementation was relatively slow, but a recent survey undertaken by Regions showed that at least 249 out of 544 posts released (46%) had been filled by the end of 1990. Regions have reported recently that they receive more requests for staff grade posts than they have approval for, indicating that the rate of uptake is continuing to improve.

There are two important aspects to the introduction of the staff grade. From the point of view of the patient it introduces an element of long-term stability of medical staffing, both in outpatient clinics and in the wards, to counterbalance the rapid turnover of doctors in training. From the postholder's point of view there are a number of doctors who wish to have a long-term clinical commitment without taking on the responsibilities of the consultant grade.

Implementation of the other measures outlined in *Achieving a Balance* is continuing at a good pace, with significant progress. The Joint Planning Advisory Committee (JPAC), whose work is an integral part of *Achieving a Balance*, determines the number of training grade doctors at the registrar and senior registrar level in each specialty. It has completed an initial scrutiny of all specialties, has recommended targets for both senior registrar and registrar grades, and has now embarked on a programme of regular reviews of all the specialties. The senior registrar scrutinies were completed first, and health authorities have been notified of their allocations. The Regional allocations for NHS career registrars were issued early in 1990[5].

Separate academic and research quotas will be issued in 1991. In addition to opportunities for those registrars able to pursue a career in the UK, there are still opportunities for overseas doctors to undertake postgraduate training as visiting registrars, and an increasing number are doing so through the overseas doctors' training schemes of several Royal Colleges.

(iii) Women doctors and their careers

The Working Party on Women Doctors and their Careers, set up in 1989 jointly by DH and the Joint Consultants Committee (JCC), continued to meet throughout 1990. It examined practical approaches to some of the issues raised by Dr Isobel Allen's earlier study on doctors and their careers[6].

Almost equal numbers of men and women qualify from medical school, but only 15% of consultants are women and in the surgical specialties the proportion is only 3%. In the view of the Working Party it is essential to tackle these anomalies if the NHS is to make full use of women doctors, who are a major asset and resource. The three main issues examined by the Working Party were:

a. Under representation of women at consultant level

The Working Party is proposing a scheme, fully supported by the RCS, to identify women undertaking training in surgical specialties to ensure that they receive support and encouragement to help them progress. It is to be called the WIST (Women in Surgical Training) scheme.

b. Opportunities for part-time working

The Working Party is making recommendations for improved and increased opportunities for part-time working for both women and men, and welcomes the introduction by DH of a new Regionally based scheme at registrar level, which will be supported by central top sliced funding.

c. Equal opportunities in appointments procedures

DH is already preparing new guidance on appointments procedures, and the Working Party contributed very helpful and detailed comments seeking to ensure that direct and indirect discrimination is eliminated.

The Working Party will be making a number of recommendations on these and other issues, in a Report due to be published early in 1991, and will be asking DH, health authorities and the Royal Colleges to take these forward.

(iv) Postgraduate and continuing medical education

On 6 July 1990, the Secretary of State announced at a joint conference on postgraduate medical education that he had accepted the recommendations of the Chief Medical Officer's Expert Advisory Group on the way postgraduate medical education should be funded and organised in the post-reform NHS. The Secretary of State outlined ten principles which the Expert Advisory Group had formulated as a guide to defining a future system for postgraduate and continuing medical education. These principles included the creation of protected budgets for postgraduate and continuing education. The budget holder for postgraduate education would be the Regional Postgraduate Dean, and for continuing education the Unit General Manager. On 12 September the

Department issued an Executive Letter outlining the new arrangements for the delivery of postgraduate and continuing medical education in Regions[7]. The letter asked Regions to identify what is currently spent on the direct costs of postgraduate and continuing education. These figures will be used to form the basis of the budgets at Regional and Unit level.

April 1990 saw the introduction of the Postgraduate Education Allowance for GPs, which is described on page 165. During the year, the Standing Committee on Postgraduate Medical Education (SCOPME) published its First Report covering its work between August 1988 and June 1990[8] and a report of *An assessment of NHS expenditure on postgraduate medical education in England in 1988/89*[9], and prepared a proposal for a new infrastructure for postgraduate medical training and continuing education.

(v) Undergraduate medical and dental education

In 1989, the Steering Group on Undergraduate Medical and Dental Education was asked to assess the implications of the proposed NHS reforms and to make recommendations. In June 1990, the Steering Group published its Second Report[10], which included 33 recommendations. The Report was endorsed by the Secretaries of State for Health and for Education and Science. High standards of medical and dental education require an environment which combines high professional standards with a spirit of intellectual enquiry based on active research and development programmes. To achieve this, the Steering Group emphasised that close and effective collaboration between universities and the NHS is essential. The Group established ten key principles which should underpin the joint working arrangements that prove most suitable; such arrangements must adhere to the ten key principles.

The arrangements for the distribution of the Service Increment for Teaching and Research (SIFTR) have been improved. In future, health authorities will collaborate with universities in setting contracts for the support the NHS will provide in return for SIFTR, which covers the excess service costs of teaching and research. Support for teaching in general practice has also been improved. In April 1990, GPs who teach medical students in their practices started receiving the Student Allowance, and in September university departments of general practice received their first payments from a new fund of £400,000 per year. A new Steering Group was established in October to monitor the impact of the NHS reforms as they are implemented. Its remit was extended to include the service implications of research.

References

1   Department of Health. *Junior doctors' hours*. Department of Health, 1990. (Executive Letter: EL(90)227).

2   Department of Health. *Heads of Agreement: Ministerial Group on Junior Doctors' Hours*. Department of Health, 1990.

3   Newton T, Grabham AH, Roberts G. *Hospital medical staffing: achieving a balance: plan for action: a report issued by the steering group for implementation on behalf of the UK Health Departments, the Joint Consultants Committee and Chairmen of Regional Health Authorities*. London: Department of Health and Social Security, 1987.

4   Department of Health. *Working for Patients: the NHS review*. London: HMSO, 1989. (Cm. 555).

5   Department of Health. *Joint planning advisory committee—definitive quotas for career registrars*. London: Department of Health, 1990. (Executive Letter: EL(90)P47).

6   Allen I. *Doctors and their careers*. London: Policy Studies Institute, 1988. (PSI research Report; 675).

7   Department of Health. Postgraduate and continuing medical and dental education. Department of Health, 1990. (Executive Letter: EL (90)179).

8   Standing Committee on Postgraduate Medical Education (SCOPME). *First report: the work of the Standing Committee on Postgraduate Medical Education: August 1988 to June 1990.* London: HMSO, 1990.

9   Standing Committee on Postgraduate Medical Education (SCOPME). *An assessment of NHS expenditure on postgraduate medical education in England in 1988/89.* London: HMSO, 1990.

10 Department of Health. *Undergraduate Medical and Dental Education: Second Report of the Steering Group.* London: Department of Health, 1990.

(g) Dental health

(i) Dental health of the Nation

The Adult Dental Health Survey of 1988, the results of which will be published early in 1991, was the third of the decennial series and, as usual, allows predictions to be made. It therefore has important implications for the practice of dentistry. Examination of some of the key indicators spanning the 20-year period between 1968 and 1988 is of considerable interest. For example, a primary goal for dental health is the avoidance of total tooth loss. In 1988, 79% of the UK adult population had some natural teeth, compared with 70% in 1978, and 63% in England and Wales in 1968. To a large extent the 1988 position reflects the historical pattern of total tooth loss. If the younger cohorts are considered, it is evident that there is very little total tooth loss in these groups. It is predicted that the population of the UK with no natural teeth will fall from 20% in 1988 to 14% in 1998, 10% in 2008, and 7% in 2018, and will come to rest at 6% in 2028.

The Survey takes an arbitrary view that the possession of 21 or more standing teeth is an indication of a functional, predominantly natural dentition, and proposed this as a readily quantifiable goal of oral health. It found that 63% of adults in the UK still had 21 or more of their own teeth in 1988, compared with 51% in 1978. It is anticipated that by 2008 at least 92% of the working-age population will have a functional dentition as defined in these terms.

Against a background in England and Wales of a population increase of 11% between 1968 and 1988, the number of dentate adults rose by 41%. The pool of natural teeth increased by 57% and the number of sound untreated teeth increased by 65%, representing a substantial improvement in dental health. Additionally, the number of filled but otherwise sound teeth rose by 72%, a tribute to the effort of the dental profession in working towards better dental health. Whilst this optimistic picture concerns all adults over the age of 16 years, the most dramatic improvements were recorded in young adults. Nevertheless, there remained a pool of 32 million decayed or unsound teeth. This, coupled with the finding that one third of dentate adults do not use the dental services unless in dire straits, indicates that there is still much for the profession to do.

The Survey also looked at attitudes to dental care, and interviews showed that, while many patients perceived the cost of treatment as a barrier, fear and negative images of dentistry and the dental practice environment were more powerful deterrents. There remains much scope for stimulating a greater uptake of services, and practitioners will need to show ingenuity in overcoming the barriers.

Figure 7.6: *Dental caries experience of 5-year-old children, Great Britain, 1988 and 1990*

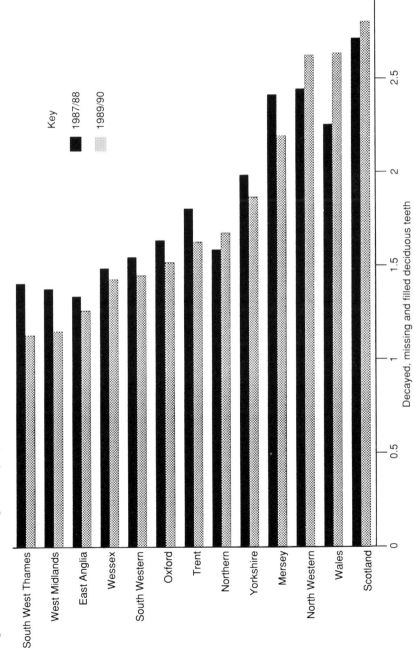

Source: Journal of Community Dentistry June 1991.

The overall picture is an encouraging one of continuing improvement in the Nation's dental health. It gives important pointers for the effective development of appropriate dental services, including a more focused reorientation towards prevention. The new contract for general dental services (GDS) should assist this process.

Children's dental health is also improving, although the caries prevalence statistics from health authorities do show significant Regional variations. For example, the mean number of decayed, missing and filled primary teeth in 5-year-old children in the North Western Region (2.64) is more than twice that in South West Thames (1.14). Comparisons by Region are illustrated in Figure 7.6. The statistics conceal some polarisation of the severity of the disease, with those children from Social Classes IIIM, IV and V, and from deprived backgrounds, having appreciably higher levels of untreated caries. There is also evidence to show that there is a high level (up to 8-10%) of rampant caries in pre-school children in some Districts.

(ii) General dental services

The major feature of 1990 was the introduction, on 1 October, of a new dental contract, the first major revision of GDS since the inception of the NHS. Patients are now offered continuing care with a written treatment plan, preventive treatment, emergency cover, and replacement of certain restorations free of charge if they fail within a year. Patients under 18 years-of-age now register with a dentist under a capitation arrangement which covers most items of treatment, including prevention. The provision of orthodontic care, surgery, general anaesthesia, items involving laboratory costs, and treatment following trauma are covered by an item of service payment system. A continuing care payment is made to dentists in respect of adult patients registered with them. By 31 December, 7,007,021 adults had registered for continuing care, and 2,380,267 children under the capitation arrangement.

The Dental Practice Board (DPB) authorised 4.4% fewer estimates in 1989/90—34,558,530 compared with 36,155,767 the previous year. The DPB considers that this fall was more apparent than real, mainly due to speedier handling of estimates at the end of 1988/89. This reduced the backlog of estimates so that significantly more were actually authorised in 1988/89 than in 1989/90. The number of dentists working in the GDS rose by 310 from 15,868 to 16,178, an increase of 2%[1].

The management of the Dental Reference Service was transferred from DH to the DPB on 15 March 1990. The Dental Officers (DOs) of the Reference Service carried out 22,181 examinations in 1990, excluding those relating to orthodontic treatment, largely at the request of the DPB. This was a fall of 4.5% compared with 1989, due to a period of uncertainty prior to the transfer, and changes in the clerical staff afterwards. In those cases for which treatment had been completed, the assessments showed 93.7% to be wholly or mainly satisfactory. Where treatment was planned, DOs were in broad agreement with 79.7% of treatment proposals.

The gross fees authorised for GDS practitioners in England and Wales rose by 0.6% from £967,407,734 to £973,003,258. Patients' contributions accounted for 39.7% of these fees, as opposed to 31.9% in 1989. This increase can be largely attributed to the introduction of patient contributions to the cost of dental examinations on 1 January 1989. Thus public funding of general dental services in England and Wales fell from £659,842,007 in 1988/89 to £587,892,773 in 1989/90, a reduction of £71,949,234 (10.9%). The average cost per estimate rose by 5.2% to £28.15. As in previous years, almost half of the cost of the GDS was attributable to conservative treatment (47.6%); periodontal treatment for adults accounted for a further 13.8%.

(iii) Community dental services

Statistical returns of the activity of the community dental services are submitted by DHAs to DH in April each year. In 1991 the returns will be on a new Körner form, KC64, and will record the levels of activity under various headings, including Preventive Programmes, Screening, Health Education and Patient Care. Previous returns, on Form 28M, concentrated on the number of inspections and types of treatment provided in various age-groups. As 1990 was the last year in which statistics in this form were received, it was therefore the last year for which comparisons with previous years were possible.

In 1989/90 the number of inspections carried out on children under 5 years-of-age fell to 216,088, 3.3% fewer than in the previous year; of these children, 40% required treatment. This proportion has been static for the last two years, supporting the belief that the decline in caries in young children is levelling out[2]. The number of inspections on schoolchildren dropped by 6.2% to 4,316,339, whereas the number of handicapped adults inspected rose by 3.6% to 84,145. The number of completed courses of treatment for this latter group rose by 7.7% to 49,629. The total number of teeth extracted in the community dental services fell by 1.5%, and the total number of general anaesthetics administered fell by 2.8% to 72,130.

The latest available figures, published in September 1989, show a fall in the total number of whole time equivalent dental officers of 8.2% compared with the previous year. However, the proportion of senior dental officers to dental officers rose from 34% in September 1988 to 40% in September 1989. All senior dental officers have special responsibilities, and often have postgraduate qualifications in specialist fields. This change in manpower ratios is one indication that the community dental services are adapting to their changed role following implementation of the Health and Medicines Act 1988[3]. The 20th Report of the Review Body on Doctors' and Dentists' Remuneration[4] recommended that Specialists in Community Dental Health should be paid on the consultant salary scale from April 1990. In November 1990, in accordance with this recommendation, the Health Departments announced that Specialists in Community Dental Health would in future be known as Consultants in Dental Public Health.

(iv) Hospital dental services

New outpatient referrals to consultant clinics in the four dental specialties rose by 5.8%, from 535,609 in 1988/89 to 566, 923 in 1989/90. Oral surgery showed the largest increase, with 393,122 people referred in 1989/90 compared with 365,064 in the previous year (a rise of 7.7%). The number of new patient referrals in restorative dentistry fell by 1.6% to 65,304, and in paediatric dentistry there was a fall of 0.9% to 17,929. Outpatient referrals to consultant orthodontic clinics rose by 5.2%, from 86,067 in 1988/89 to 90,568 in 1989/90. The total number of consultant initiated outpatient attendances (repeat attendances) showed a slight fall of 0.27% to 614,670 in 1989/90 compared with the previous year. The number of scheduled operating theatre sessions in oral surgery held in the year ending 31 March 1990 was 32,763, a rise of 453 (1.4%) compared with the previous year. The total number of cases operated on in these and other sessions rose by 3,915 (3.1%) to 131,049[5,6].

(v) Continuing education and training for dentists

The voluntary vocational training scheme for the GDS, which commenced in 1988, has continued to expand. By December 1990 there were 309 trainees divided between 33 Regionally based programmes. If vocational training becomes mandatory, it is estimated that 520 places in 44 programmes will be required.

The Committee for Continuing Education and Training (COCET) identified the following topics as priority areas for postgraduate training in 1990: minimal intervention techniques and the use of modern materials; the problems of the ageing dentition; the training of trainers; opportunities for change and evolution arising from the new contract; health and safety at work; courses to reinforce the video training programme; the involvement of dentists in the Teamwork Project; and 'hands on' courses on a variety of topics. The Regional Postgraduate Deans organised these courses under section 63[7] in addition to arranging training locally for dental practitioners, including hospital and community service dentists. Under the provisions of the National Health Service and Community Care Act 1990, the role of Postgraduate Dental Deans was enhanced by the allocation of budgets for continuing education.

The programme of training videos continued in 1990, and five more titles were completed and distributed. These were: *Adhesive Dentistry,* which relates to the use of composite and glass ionomer filling materials in conservative dentistry; *Adding Life to Years*, which deals with the management of elderly patients; *Emergency in the Dental Surgery*, which describes resuscitation techniques; *Capitation*, which introduces the concept of continuing care for children through the experiences of dentists who had taken part in the capitation trials; and a video to accompany training notes for the introduction of the new contract.

The Masterclass initiative was launched in May 1990, in collaboration with the British Dental Association. This project is designed to help dentists and their staff communciate with patients and each other in a more effective manner. The Teamwork project also started in 1990, and will continue throughout 1991. This is a collaborative project with the British Dental Journal; it is designed to help dentists train their Dental Surgery Assistants within the practice environment, using a series of journal articles with supporting material and local seminars.

(vi) Dental research

The elderly

The elderly represent an increasing proportion of the population and many more elderly people are retaining some of their natural dentition into advancing years. The dental status, needs and demands of this group of people are unclear, but more individuals are presenting for dental care with complex management problems, including tooth wear, periodontal disease and root surface caries.

The University of Newcastle Upon Tyne Dental School has been commissioned to undertake a study of the dental status, needs and demands of samples of the elderly population from the North and South of England. It is proposed to examine 2,400 individuals over a 3-year period.

Oral health education

During 1990 DH funded a variety of experimental oral health education projects, in Dudley, Sefton, South Tyneside, Derbyshire and the North Western Region. On 28 November 1990 DH held an oral health education seminar entitled *The Way Forward*. During the seminar the results of recent experimental projects and surveys were presented, and strategies for the future discussed.

General anaesthesia

The Report of an Expert Working Party under the chairmanship of Professor David Poswillo was published in March 1990[8]. The Group was established following the recommendation of the Standing Dental Advisory Committee; its terms of reference were "To examine and make recommendations with regard to all aspects of general anaesthesia, sedation and resuscitation in dentistry outside hospitals". The Report emphasises the need to avoid the use of general anaesthesia wherever possible, and to persuade patients of the benefits of alternative techniques. It has been issued for consultation to representative groups within the dental and medical professions.

References

1 Dental Practice Board. *Annual Report 1989/90*. Eastbourne: Dental Practice Board, 1990.

2 Downer MC. Time trends in decay in young children. *Health Trends* 1989; **21**: 7-9.

3 *Health and Medicines Act 1988*. London: HMSO, 1988.

4 Review Body on Doctors' & Dentists' Remuneration. *Twentieth report*. London: HMSO, 1990. Chairman: Sir Graham Wilkins. (Cm. 937).

5 Department of Health. *NHS operating theatres availability and use 1988/89*. London: Department of Health, 1990.

6 *Department of Health. NHS operating theatres availability and use 1989/90*. London: Department of Health, 1990.

7 *Health Services and Public Health Act 1968*. London: HMSO, 1968.

8 Standing Dental Advisory Committee. *General anaesthesia, sedation and resuscitation in dentistry: Report of an Expert Working Party*. London: Department of Health, 1990.

8. CONTROL OF MEDICINES, ENVIRONMENTAL HEALTH AND TOXICOLOGY

(a) Medicines Control Agency

(i) Reorganisation

The reorganisation of the Medicines Control Agency (MCA) into multi-disciplinary functional units, as recommended by Mr Cunliffe and Dr Evans in their *Study into the Control of Medicines*[1], was successfully implemented in 1990.

The Agency, although remaining part of the Department of Health (DH), is now managed by a Director, supported by six functional business managers and a finance director selected for their managerial ability as well as their technical expertise. These managers are in turn supported by Group Managers and co-ordinators who are responsible for the co-ordination of multidisciplinary units. The Agency's Director currently reports to a Deputy Secretary on management issues and a Deputy Chief Medical Officer on medical issues. These reporting lines will disappear when the Agency becomes an Executive Agency in 1991.

The MCA has a major professional and technical component to its function, and the management reorganisation has, therefore, been supplemented by posts recognising the important professional contribution in areas outside line management. The appointees have been designated as principal professional assessors to the Licensing Authority's advisory bodies and their sub-committees, and these posts represent alternative career pathways for those of the Agency's highly trained and very valuable professional staff who do not have an interest in line management responsibilities.

(ii) Developments in the European Community

One of the MCA's functions is to provide advice on international licensing matters affecting medicinal products for human use. Activity in the European Community (EC) during 1990 showed a marked increase as the 1992 deadline for completion of the single market, which includes pharmaceuticals, approached.

Rational use Directives

In January, three draft Directives were presented by the European Commission. The first provides for specific authorisation for wholesale dealers and for controls on the wholesale distribution of medicines to retail level, and largely reflects current United Kingdom (UK) practice. The second Directive sets out common criteria for determining whether or not a medicine should be available on a prescription only basis. The third in this series aims to harmonise and improve the information provided to patients and health care professionals. The UK welcomed the objectives behind the proposals, but had reservations on some points of detail, on which negotiations continue.

Homoeopathic products

In March, the Commission published proposals to bring homoeopathic medicinal products within the scope of community law. These were specifically excluded from earlier Directives governing medicinal products in the EC. The proposals open options for a simplified registration system without a requirement to demonstrate efficacy for some homoeopathic products. Discussion of these proposals is expected in 1991.

Advertising

In June, the Commission put forward a draft Directive providing for a common framework for, and introducing controls on, advertising medicines to the public and the professions. This proposal has caused concern about the possible impact on existing arrangements in the UK for the monitoring of advertisements and promotional activities, and, in particular, on the industry's sponsorship of genuine educational programmes, seminars and conferences. Discussions on this proposal are scheduled to start early in 1991.

Future European Community licensing systems

Following a prolonged and extensive consultation, the Commission undertook a major review of licensing arrangements in the EC; it culminated in a series of proposals for future systems. An important feature of these proposals is the establishment of a European Medicines Evaluation Agency to act as a central EC regulatory authority responsible for evaluating important new medicines. Most other medicines will be dealt with under the 'decentralised' procedure, which relies on the principle of mutual recognition by Member States of each other's marketing authorisations. If there is disagreement between Member States, the central Agency will provide procedures for binding arbitration. Officials are examining the implications of the proposals and are consulting widely. Phased implementation from 1 January 1993 is proposed. Discussions are at a very early stage, and the Commission is still working on the underlying technical detail in consultation with the EC Committee for Proprietary Medicinal Products.

Reference

1   Evans NJB, Cunliffe PW. *Study into the control of medicines*. Stanmore: Department of Health and Social Security, 1987.

(b) Chemical and physical agents in the environment

(i) Air pollution episodes

During recent years concern has been expressed that, although in Western countries general levels of air pollution are markedly lower than in the past, episodic air pollution might be having an adverse effect on health. This concern has been coupled with the increasing perception that air pollution is not solely a winter problem (as exemplified by the smogs in London during the 1950s), but that high levels of oxidant pollutants may be produced during fine, warm summer weather. It is generally agreed that ozone is the most important of the 'summer pollutants'.

Ozone, a secondary pollutant, is produced as a result of complex photochemical reactions from a mixture of primary pollutants (particularly the oxides of nitrogen) and atmospheric oxygen; the reactions are catalysed by volatile hydrocarbons. These complex reactions take place during the drift of air masses away from the sources of the primary pollutants (areas of high vehicle density and industrial areas), while within busy streets some of the ozone is scavenged by one of the pollutants present in vehicle exhausts, nitric oxide. This explains the apparent contradiction, which is certainly not widely understood by the public, that ozone levels are usually higher in the country than close to busy streets and roads in towns.

Ozone levels in the UK are monitored at 17 sites. The majority of these sites are located in rural areas, where ozone levels would be expected to be highest. The Warren Spring Laboratory at Stevenage is responsible for 11 of the 17 sites and monitors these telemetrically. As data are collated they are compared with the guidelines set out by WHO[1]. These guidelines incorporate a margin of safety below levels known to have adverse effects on health, but levels exceeding the guidelines are reported automatically to the Department of the Environment (DOE) and DH.

The WHO guidelines for ozone are frequently exceeded in most European countries during the summer. In the UK in the year ending March 1990, the average number of hours at the monitoring sites during which the recorded ozone concentration was in excess of 76 parts per billion (the lower end of the WHO guideline range) was 51.

In many parts of the world the background level of ozone has been shown to be higher than in the UK, and episodes of elevated ozone concentration more frequent. Los Angeles stands out as an example. In the UK the most severe episodes of elevated ozone concentration arise, in occasional years, from the drift of increasingly polluted air across industrial areas of Europe before it reaches this country. During recent years steps to reduce the production of ozone precursors have been taken by the UK and other European countries by tightening the emission standards for motor vehicles. The requirement for all new cars sold after 1993 to be fitted with three-way catalytic converters will lead to a further improvement.

It has been demonstrated that exposure to concentrations of ozone such as those experienced in the UK during episodes of pollution during the summer may produce small, temporary changes in indices of lung function. Furthermore, some workers have suggested that transient exposures to mixtures of pollutants might be playing a role in increasing the likelihood of asthmatic attacks, or of people developing asthma de novo.

In order to assess the likely effects of exposures to elevated concentrations of ozone and the main winter pollutants occurring in the UK, and whether any advice should be given to individuals to enable them to reduce their exposures to ozone, DH established the Advisory Group on Medical Aspects of Air

Pollution Episodes under the chairmanship of Professor Stephen Holgate. It has given priority to ozone, and expects to report on it in April 1991.

The Group will go on to consider other pollutants, including sulphur dioxide and acid aerosols. These pollutants are no longer the serious risk to health in the UK that they were before implementation of the Clean Air Act 1956[2], but the Group will consider whether there are any circumstances in this country in which sensitive individuals should be advised to take steps to reduce their exposure.

(ii) Health Advisory Group on Chemical Contamination Incidents

In October 1990, the Parliamentary Under Secretary of State for Health announced that the Chief Medical Officer had invited three physicians with special expertise to form an independent Health Advisory Group on Chemical Contamination Incidents, to advise Directors of Public Health (DsPH) and himself in the event of any future incident leading to chemical contamination of the water supply which might be of serious concern on health grounds. The Group will provide advice on:

– the extent to which illness occurring in the area following an incident is attributable to the toxic properties of the contaminating chemicals;

– the likelihood of prolonged or delayed health effects;

– any diagnostic or therapeutic measures which should be offered to those affected, or to the whole population of the area;

– any epidemiological or clinical investigations required to determine the nature and extent of exposure of members of the public, body burdens of pollutants, and effects; and

– any long-term health surveillance required.

The Chairman of the Advisory Group is Professor Sir Eric Stroud, formerly Professor of Child Health at King's College School of Medicine and Dentistry, and until recently Chairman of the Department's Standing Medical Advisory Committee. The epidemiologist on the Group is Dr Paul Elliot, Deputy Director of the Small Area Health Statistics Unit at the London School of Hygiene and Tropical Medicine. The third member is a clinical toxicologist, Dr Alexander Proudfoot, Director of the Scottish Poisons Information Bureau in Edinburgh, who also serves on the Advisory Committee on Pesticides and chairs its Scientific Sub-Committee.

This core group will be assisted by a panel whose members' expertise covers the wide range of scientific issues that are most likely to arise from an incident of serious chemical contamination. The Chairman will be able to call upon members according to the nature of the incident. The Advisory Group will also be supported by the Poisons Information Service. There are a number of Poisons Information Centres throughout the country, and they hold information on the toxic effects of a wide range of substances and on recommended methods of diagnosis and treatment. Access to that information is available to doctors 24 hours-a-day. DH is now planning the developments needed in the Poisons Information Service in order to cover more fully the types of chemicals that could be involved in contamination incidents, and to further improve the exchange of information between centres.

(iii) Small Area Health Statistics Unit

The Small Area Health Statistics Unit (SAHSU) is an independent body funded jointly by DH, DOE, the Health and Safety Executive (HSE) and the Scottish, Welsh and Northern Ireland Offices. It was established in 1987 at the London School of Hygiene and Tropical Medicine in order to implement one of the recommendations of the Independent Advisory Group set up under the chairmanship of Sir Douglas Black to investigate the possible increased incidence of cancer in West Cumbria. Its principal objectives are:

- to investigate possible links between pollution from industrial installations and ill health in the community; and

- to develop methods for analysing and interpreting health statistics relating to small areas (down to post code level).

SAHSU spent most of the first three years on the somewhat daunting task of building up a comprehensive data base in close collaboration with the Office of Population Censuses and Surveys and the Information and Statistics Division of the Scottish Home and Health Department. This included the distribution of mortality by specific cause, and the incidence of different types of cancer throughout the UK. In both cases information is available down to post code level.

By the autumn of 1990 the Unit was in a position to investigate rapidly reports of ill health around industrial installations. If provided with map co-ordinates, the Unit can now report on rates of cancer and mortality by age and sex within circles of varying diameter drawn from the point source. It can also give advice on whether the results of a study indicate the need for further in-depth investigation. The matter can then be referred to the appropriate expert advisory committee (eg, in the case of environmental radiation, to the Committee on Medical Aspects of Radiation in the Environment) for definitive advice on the causal agent. The first study undertaken by SAHSU related to an alleged increase in the incidence of cancer of the larynx. It involved the population in the vicinity of a small incinerator for waste oils and solvents at Charnock Richard, Lancashire. SAHSU concluded that it was unlikely that the slight increase in the ratio of observed to expected cases was associated with the incinerator. However, as a further check the study has been extended to include other incinerators of a similar type.

In addition to the rapid investigation of allegations of ill health in the vicinity of point sources of pollution, SAHSU is undertaking a long-term programme of work. It has been agreed, for example, that the Unit will investigate, at the request of DOE, the incidence of mortality and cancer in the neighbourhood of the following sites: benzene works, municipal waste incinerators, vinyl chloride works, coke works and smokeless fuel plants. These industrial operations were selected for study because they are from time to time the subject of public concern regarding the effects of pollution, and the potential of the chemicals involved to cause ill health. The information obtained will assist DOE to assess the effectiveness of current controls and to develop future policy. The results of these investigations will be published.

SAHSU is continuing to work with those involved in various cancer registries to build up background information on the distribution of disease in small areas. Initially the Unit is concentrating on the geographic distribution of leukaemias to assist in the interpretation of the significance of reported clusters of this disease. It will then progress to look at other diseases.

(iv) Leukaemia clusters and nuclear installations

In February 1990 the Medical Research Council (MRC) Environmental Epidemiology Unit at Southampton University published the results of its case control study of leukaemia and lymphoma among young people near the Sellafield nuclear plant in West Cumbria[3]. This study had been commissioned by DH in 1984 following a recommendation of the Independent Advisory Group, chaired by Sir Douglas Black[4]. It documented associations between the excess of leukaemia and non-Hodgkin's lymphoma in children, and employment of fathers in the local nuclear, iron and steel, chemical and farming industries. More particularly, it found an association between childhood leukaemia or non-Hodgkin's lymphoma and recorded level of external radiation dose received by fathers prior to conception.

The Government noted the results of the study with concern. The Parliamentary Under Secretary of State for Health referred the study to the independent expert advisory Committee on Medical Aspects of Radiation in the Environment (COMARE) for urgent consideration and advice. COMARE's advice was published in April 1990[5]. It agreed with the broad thrust of the study's main conclusions, but commented that "the important conclusions of this study are unavoidably based on very small numbers and, as these are novel observations which have not been recorded previously, we are cautious in their interpretation". COMARE stressed that causal mechanisms had not yet been identified. The Committee went on to outline possible causative mechanisms not necessarily involving ionising radiation. It stated that the study supported the case for further investigation of factors related to occupation.

COMARE recommended that other case control studies, suggested in its 2nd and 3rd Reports[6,7], should be given high priority. The Committee also recommended a further study of the health of children of radiation workers, and a study linking records of all radiation workers with national records of childhood cancer and leukaemia. The former is now under way, and a feasibility study of database linkage between the Childhood Cancer Research Group and the National Register of Radiation Workers is being undertaken. COMARE advised that further biological research was required to investigate possible causative mechanisms. The Committee then stated that it did not wish to see multiple independent studies which would cause undue inconvenience to the small numbers of individuals and families concerned. It therefore made a third recommendation: that there needed to be some form of co-ordination of research to ensure appropriate targeting of resources and to prevent unnecessary duplication of effort.

(v) Co-ordination of research on health aspects of radiation

In his announcement of COMARE's advice on the study by Gardner et al[3], the Parliamentary Under Secretary of State for Health outlined the Government's response to the specific recommendations[5]. To implement the third recommendation, DH and the HSE established an inter-departmental group—the Co-ordinating Committee on Health Aspects of Radiation Research (CCHARR). The establishment of this group also took account of a recommendation of COMARE's 2nd Report[6], that further laboratory research be undertaken to assess the importance of pre-conception fetal and early childhood exposure to ionising radiation in leukaemogenesis.

CCHARR comprises representatives from the MRC, the National Radiological Protection Board (NRPB), the United Kingdom Co-ordinating Committee on Cancer Research, and other Government Departments with an interest in this area. The Committee's terms of reference are:

- To co-ordinate relevant Government-sponsored research on the possible association between radiation and/or other factors and childhood leukaemogenesis, with reference to research nation-wide; and to maintain contact with other research co-ordination bodies, as appropriate.

- To minimise the number of multiple approaches to individuals and families arising out of such research, whether funded by Government or otherwise. To this end, the Committee will offer a 'clearing house' mechanism to alert prospective researchers to existing studies or proposals which could result in such multiple approaches.

- Within the research strategy recommended by COMARE, to invite relevant new research proposals for Government funding; to assess, with advice from independent experts, their scientific merit with reference to other research projects either under way or planned, whether funded by Government or otherwise; and to take forward relevant Government sponsored research.

As part of the 'clearing house' mechanism, CCHARR proposes to compile a register of existing and planned research projects which may be relevant to the Committee's field of activity. Information supplied or obtained for this purpose would be on a voluntary basis, and would consist solely of facts about research areas—not individuals.

(vi) Radon in the home

Radon in the home is the main source of human exposure to ionising radiation. Epidemiological studies of uranium and other miners have shown that inhalation of radon decay products can increase the risk of developing lung cancer. The average concentration of radon gas in homes in the UK is 20 Becquerels per cubic metre of air (Bq/m^3), but the levels in some homes can reach 5,000

Bq/m³. NRPB has estimated that exposure to radon at a concentration of 20 Bq/m³ corresponds to an annual radiation dose of 1 millisievert (mSv).

NRPB first issued a statement on this matter in 1987[8]. In that statement it advised that domestic exposure to radon daughters (the common name for the decay products) should be limited. An action level of 20 mSv per annum (400 Bq/m³) was recommended and accepted by the Government. It was recognised, however, that this recommendation would require regular review. NRPB recently considered new data concerning exposure to radon and its decay products, and concluded that the resultant risk of developing lung cancer is higher than previously thought. In January 1990, a statement of advice was published in which a new action level of 200 Bq/m³ was recommended[9]. It specified that areas of the UK in which 1% or more of homes exceed the action level should be regarded as 'Affected Areas'.

This advice was endorsed by COMARE, and accepted by the Government. Householders in high-risk areas have been advised that the levels of radon in their homes can be tested free of charge by NRPB on behalf of the Government. If the level is found to be above the action level, householders are advised on remedial measures to reduce it. Subsequently, in November 1990, NRPB published the results of its radon measurements in Devon and Cornwall[10]. Mapping of these results indicated that the whole of the two counties should be regarded as an 'Affected Area'. Both NRPB and COMARE have undertaken to keep this matter under review and to advise the Government if a need for further action becomes apparent.

References

1   World Health Organization. Regional office for Europe. *Air quality guidelines for Europe*. Copenhagen: World Health Organization, 1987. (WHO Regional publications: European Series; No 23).

2   *Clean Air Act 1956*. London: HMSO, 1956.

3   Gardner MJ et al. Results of a case-control study of leukaemia and lymphoma among young people near the Sellafield nuclear plant in West Cumbria. *Br Med J* 1990; **300**: 423–9.

4   *Investigation of the possible increased incidence of cancer in West Cumbria. Report of the Independent Advisory Group*. London: HMSO, 1984. Chairman: Sir Douglas Black.

5   House of Commons. Parliamentary Debate. Radiation: Committee on the Medical Aspects of Radiation in the Environment. *Hansard* 2 April 1990; **170**: Col 430-34(w).

6   Committee on Medical Aspects of Radiation in the Environment (COMARE). *Second Report. Investigation of the possible increased incidence of childhood cancer in the vicinity of the Dounreay Nuclear Establishment, Caithness, Scotland*. London: HMSO, 1988.

7   Committee on Medical Aspects of Radiation in the Environment (COMARE). *Third Report. Report on the Incidence of Childhood Cancer in the West Berkshire and North Hampshire area, in which are situated the Atomic Weapons Research Establishment, Aldermaston and the Royal Ordnance Factory, Burghfield*. London: HMSO, 1989.

8   National Radiological Protection Board. *Exposure to radon daughters in dwellings*. London: HMSO, 1987. (Series ASP 10).

9   National Radiological Protection Board. Board statement on radon in homes. *Documents of the NRPB* 1990; **1**(1): 15-32.

10 National Radiological Protection Board. Radon affected areas: Cornwall and Devon. *Documents of the NRPB* 1990; **1**(4): 35-43.

(c) Toxicological safety

(i) Vitamin A

It has become apparent that pregnant women can obtain excess quantities of vitamin A from supplements and liver, in addition to the essential levels present in a normal balanced diet. Since there is sufficient published evidence to conclude that vitamin A is probably a low-grade teratogen in humans[1], there is the possibility that fetuses may be at risk. There have been concerns about excessive intakes of vitamin A by pregnant women[2,3,4,5], and expert bodies have expressed the view that a reasonable upper limit for total vitamin A intake during the first three months of pregnancy, the period during which the embryo and fetus are most at risk, is 3,300 micrograms daily. In view of these concerns, the question of vitamin A intake during pregnancy was referred to the Committee on the Toxicity of Chemicals in Food, Consumer Products and the Environment (COT).

COT was aware that some pregnant women are already given vitamin supplements as part of their ante-natal care. The amount of vitamin A given under medical supervision is carefully chosen to provide that amount necessary for the health of the mother and child, while avoiding any possibility of ill effects. However, the Committee considered that pregnant women, or women who may become pregnant, should be advised against additional self-medication with dietary supplements containing vitamin A. The majority of vitamin supplements now available on retail sale do not contain more than 750 micrograms of vitamin A in any individual dose. Any supplements of vitamin A containing amounts greater than 750 micrograms should carry a warning specifically directed to pregnant women stating that they should not be taken unless medical advice has been obtained.

COT considered that some samples of liver contained very high levels of vitamin A, and that the levels in a normal serving of a 100 gram portion were above those regarded as healthy for the developing fetus. They also recognised that for many years levels in some livers have probably been high. Since the critical period for adverse effects is in the early weeks of pregnancy, and women cannot know whether they are eating liver with a vitamin A content at these exceptionally high levels, COT recommended that, as a matter of prudence, women who are pregnant or may become pregnant should refrain from eating liver or liver products for the time being.

The Committee took care to point out that there is currently no evidence that any birth defects have occurred in the UK as a result of vitamin A intakes. However, there have been a small number of case reports from abroad of birth defects in children of women who have taken supplements containing vitamin A greatly in excess of the recommended daily amount. World-wide there has been only one case reported of birth defects thought to have been due to the consumption of liver in pregnancy. In this case the woman had consumed large quantities of liver every day during her pregnancy.

In October 1990 the Chief Medical Officer advised women who are pregnant, or who might become pregnant, not to take excessive quantities of vitamin A.

(ii) L-tryptophan

The Report for 1989[6] described the appearance in the USA of a new clinical syndrome, Eosinophilia-Myalgia Syndrome (EMS). This syndrome was associated with the use of food supplement products containing the amino-acid L-tryptophan. Over 1,500 cases, including 27 deaths, have been reported in the

USA. During 1990, 16 possible cases of EMS in the UK were reported to DH. Five of these were associated with the use of food supplements, and 11 with the use of prescription medicines containing L-tryptophan[7]. These medicines were withdrawn from general use by the manufacturers in April 1990 and doctors were informed in a letter from the Chairman of the Committee on Safety of Medicines.

In November 1989, DH advised that the sale of food supplement products in which L-tryptophan is the sole or major ingredient should cease, and that such products should not be imported. However, during 1990 it became clear that these products were still being sold, and that the syndrome could be provoked by the ingestion of small amounts of added tryptophan. Therefore, in August 1990, Regulations banning the addition of tryptophan to food, and the sale of food containing added tryptophan unless it is needed on medical grounds, were made[8].

Following investigations by the US Food and Drug Administration, it has become clear that most cases of EMS are associated with L-tryptophan from a single source in Japan produced by a fermentation process employing a genetically modified bacterium. The cause of the syndrome is unknown, but it may be a contaminant produced in the fermentation process. Studies to identify the contaminant concerned are under way in the USA.

(iii) Cling film and other packaging materials

Plastic packaging materials, including cling film, for wrapping foods play an important role in reducing contamination of food by harmful micro-organisms. Nevertheless, it is necessary to consider alongside such benefits other health aspects, such as the extent to which chemicals migrate from packaging materials into foods and beverages, and whether this might pose any risk to health.

Analysis of foods and beverages to detect chemicals migrating from packaging materials is carried out by the Ministry of Agriculture, Fisheries and Food (MAFF), as part of an ongoing surveillance programme which has been under way for a number of years[9,10]. For example, plasticisers, which give flexibility and can impart cling properties to plastic food packaging materials, have been studied in depth because they can migrate in significant amounts, especially into fatty foods and into foods being heated[11,12]. The findings of the surveillance programme are regularly reviewed by COT. In its most recent advice[11], COT welcomed the reductions in intake of the plasticiser di-2-ethylhexyl adipate (DEHA) which have occurred since the previous review[12], but expressed concern about the increasing use of other plasticisers on which there is very little toxicological information. COT emphasised that any substances proposed for use in food packaging materials and which are likely to give rise to an appreciable intake should not be utilised until appropriate toxicological testing and evaluation have been carried out.

In view of COT's concerns, MAFF's Food Advisory Committee recommended that consumers should be advised not to use cling films in conventional ovens, or for wrapping food or lining dishes when cooking in a microwave oven. It also advised that cling films should not be used for wrapping foods with a high fat content, such as cheese. This advice was issued by MAFF in November

1990[13,14] as a precautionary measure while additional work is carried out to provide the necessary toxicological information on some of the plasticisers in use.

(iv) Lead in cattle feed

In November 1989, cattle feed contaminated with lead was inadvertently imported into the UK and widely distributed to cattle and dairy farms. Nearly 1,500 farms, located mainly in the South West of England, received contaminated feed. Prompt action by DH and MAFF prevented lead contaminated food from entering the food chain.

It has been the policy of successive Governments since 1974 to contain and reduce lead exposure wherever practicable[15]. Animals identified by blood tests as having eaten contaminated feed were confined to farms, and not allowed to be sent for slaughter. In those dairy farms where lead contaminated feed had been eaten, strict limits on the concentrations of lead allowable in milk were imposed. Milk containing in excess of these levels was sequestrated and not released into the food chain. Continuous monitoring of the milk obtained from contaminated herds showed rapid decline in lead levels after the cows were switched to normal feed.

Meat, bone and offal, particularly liver and kidney, were more problematical. It has long been known that lead concentrates in bone, liver and kidney. When analysed, bone showed high concentrations of lead. Initially, therefore, meat that met the stringent lead requirements coud be sold only off the bone. Experiments soon showed that bone lead was virtually irreversibly sequestered under a variety of common cooking conditions, and posed a negligible health risk. In addition, there was the added safety factor that bones are not generally eaten. Thereafter, meat conforming to the low lead levels was allowed to be sold on the bone. Liver and kidney were the final products allowed back on to the market. They were initially destroyed, and only released when serial sampling revealed that their lead levels had diminished sufficiently to conform to the Lead in Food Regulations 1979[16].

Although a large number of farms and approximately 110,000 animals were involved, continuous monitoring of lead levels in all foodstuffs, together with close co-operation between DH and MAFF, ensured that at no time did any foodstuff pose a risk to health.

(v) Expert Working Group on Sudden Infant Death Syndrome

In March 1990 the Chief Medical Officer announced the establishment of an Expert Working Group[17] to investigate Mr Barry Richardson's hypothesis that a cause of Sudden Infant Death Syndrome (SIDS) was the liberation of phosphine, stibine or arsine by the action of the mould *Scopulariopsis brevicaulis* on compounds present in PVC used in cot mattress covers. Limited experimental evidence was provided to support the generation of such toxic gases by microbial action.

The Group was chaired by Professor Paul Turner. At its first meeting certain experimental studies were identified as being essential before any conclusions could be reached. These involved investigating the potential for gas formation, using specific and quantitative methods under optimum laboratory conditions. In addition, there was a need for similar studies on samples obtained from cot deaths and handled under controlled conditions to avoid adventitious contamination. An extensive programme of collaborative work was agreed between the Laboratory of the Government Chemist (LGC) and the International Mycological Institute (IMI), Kew. This was funded jointly by DH and the Department of Trade and Industry, and was completed in October 1990.

In the meantime, the Expert Working Group considered information from many organisations and individuals. The main aspects covered were:

- The unequivocal identification and quantification of any evolved gases from the antimony and phosphorus compounds present in PVC.

- The epidemiology of SIDS and any relationship between time trends and changes in cot mattress materials.

- The toxicity of any of the gases that could potentially be evolved.

It became clear during the investigation that Mr Richardson's experimental work could not be replicated by the LGC and others. In addition, the procedures he used were not specific for a given toxic gas, nor were they quantitative. The absence of precautions against microbial contamination was also noted. Other findings were that there was no direct pathological evidence to link SIDS to the generation of such toxic gases. This observation, by itself, did not invalidate the hypothesis as no data on the reaction of infants to such toxic gases were available. It was also considered pertinent that the incidence of SIDS had remained remarkably consistent since its recognition as a cause of death. This mitigated against the toxic gas hypothesis being a cause of more than a very small proportion of SIDS cases. A finding incidental to the main investigation was microbial contamination of cot mattresses, and the significance of this finding is being assessed.

The detailed report of the LGC/IMI work was considered at the last meeting of the Working Group in November 1990. Its report, which concluded that Mr Richardson's hypothesis was not supported by experimental evidence, was finalised by the end of the year. The Working Group made a number of recommendations relating to the toxicity and purity of the antimony and phosphorus compounds used in cot furnishings. In addition, the need for further work on the significance of the microbial contamination, and the need to consider a British Standard for resistance of cot mattresses to such contamination, were noted.

Note: The report was published in June 1991.

References

1   Bielsalski HK. Comparative assessment of the toxicology of vitamin A and retinoids in man. *Toxicology* 1990; **57**: 117-61.
2   Teratology Society Position Paper. Vitamin A during pregnancy: Recommendations for vitamin A supplementation during pregnancy. *Teratology* 1987; **35**: 268.
3   The American College of Obstetricians and Gynaecologists (ACOG). *ACOG Committee Statement; Vitamin A supplementation during pregnancy.* One East Wacker Drive, Suite 2700, Chicago (Illinois), 1987.

4 Council for Responsible Nutrition (CRN). Vitamin A policy. *CRN News* 1987; 1-2, 2100 M Street, NW, Suite 602, Washington DC.

5 International Vitamin A Consultative Group (IVACG). *Position Paper: The safe use of vitamin A by women during the reproductive years*. 1986 (April). IVACG Secretariat, ILSI, 1126 Sixteenth Street, NW, Washington DC.

6 Department of Health. *On the State of the Public Health: the annual report of the Chief Medical Officer of the Department of Health for the year 1989*. London: HMSO, 1990; 146.

7 Committee on Safety of Medicines. *Current Problems, Number 29*. August 1990.

8 *Tryptophan in Food Regulations 1990*. London: HMSO, 1990.

9 Ministry of Agriculture, Fisheries and Food. *The surveillance of food contamination in the United Kingdom: the first report of the Steering Group on Food Surveillance*. London: HMSO, 1978.

10 Ministry of Agriculture, Fisheries and Food. *Food surveillance 1985 to 1988: the twenty-fourth report of the Steering Group on Food Surveillance*. London: HMSO, 1988.

11 Ministry of Agriculture, Fisheries and Food. *Plasticisers: continuing surveillance: the thirtieth report of the Steering Group on Food Surveillance*. London: HMSO, 1990.

12 Ministry of Agriculture, Fisheries and Food. *Survey of plasticiser levels in food contact materials and in foods: the twenty-first report of the Steering Group on Food Surveillance*. London: HMSO, 1987.

13 Ministry of Agriculture, Fisheries and Food. *Extensive information on food wrapping published*. News Release 12 November 1990. MAFF, Whitehall Place, London SW1A 2HH.

14 Ministry of Agriculture, Fisheries and Food. *Cling films*. Food Safety Directorate Information. Issue Number 7.1 November 1990. MAFF, Public Enquiry Point, Room 303a, Ergon House, c/o Nobel House, 17 Smith Square, London SW1P 3JR.

15 *Lead in Food: Progress Report. The twenty-seventh report of the Steering Group on Food Surveillance: The Working Party on Inorganic Contaminants in Food: Third Supplementary report on lead*. London: HMSO, 1989.

16 *Lead in Food Regulations*. London: HMSO, 1979. (Statutory Instrument 1641).

17 Department of Health. *Independent experts to review possible link between cot deaths and toxic gases*. London: Department of Health, 1990. (Press Release 90/118).

9. INTERNATIONAL HEALTH

(a) Britain, Europe and health

The importance to Britain of developments in the health sector in Europe grew steadily throughout 1990. These included developments within the European Community (EC) on control of pharmaceuticals and medical devices, safety of food, mutual recognition of professional qualifications, and research and development—all subjects which fall within the scope of the Treaties establishing the European Communities. Health Ministers, acting partly as an EC Council, and partly as representatives of the governments of Member States, also increased their activities. At the end of the year the European summit meeting agreed that health should be included among the subjects to be considered in the Inter-Governmental Conference on Political Union for specific inclusion within the Treaty. The Community also made important contributions to the Central European States under the Poland and Hungary Assistance for Economic Restructuring (PHARE) programme and, by extension of its programmes, to the former German Democratic Republic as part of a unified Germany.

WHO was also active in Central Europe, making emergency contributions of medical supplies and launching programmes of assistance. The United Kingdom (UK) contributions included the grant of £500,000 to a WHO emergency fund for Rumania. In addition, WHO established a centre for Environment and Health on two sites, respectively in the Netherlands and in Italy, to be guided by the advice of a scientific committee chaired by Sir Donald Acheson in his personal capacity. A nutrition conference was held in Budapest, and a conference on demand reduction in drug abuse was held in London. WHO's 'Health for All by the Year 2000' programme underwent a further evaluation, and its approach assisted work on a health strategy for this country.

The Council of Europe undertook further work on bioethics, and held a Health Ministers' conference on health manpower.

(b) European Community—co-operation on health matters

(i) The Health Council

The Health Ministers, meeting in Council on 17 May 1990 under the Irish Presidency, adopted the 2nd Action Programme against Cancer. No consensus of opinion was reached on restrictions on the advertising of tobacco products and the draft Directive was referred for further discussion. The Council also discussed and approved Presidency Communications on Action Against Drugs, AIDS, Youth and Health, and the rational use of medicinal products.

On 3 December 1990, the Council, under the Italian Presidency, adopted draft Council Resolutions on Nutrition, and Health and Doping in Sport. Draft Conclusions on the Safety of Food, Drink and Water for Human Consumption, Drugs and AIDS were all approved. Under the Action Programme against Cancer, the draft Directive on Advertising of Tobacco Products, which had been considered at earlier Health Councils, was again discussed, but the necessary majority was not reached. It was therefore withdrawn. The Commission intend to submit a further proposal. Commission communications on health protection, EC/WHO co-operation, biomedical research, and a future system for a European Licensing system for medicinal products were also discussed.

(ii) Smoking

Tobacco labelling

Draft Regulations to implement the EC Tobacco Products Labelling Directive, adopted at the end of 1989, will be published for consultation early in 1991. The regulations will introduce new, stronger health warnings to be displayed prominently on all tobacco products.

Advertising

A number of Member States, including the UK, had reservations on the draft EC Directive on tobacco advertising and, at their meeting in December 1990, EC Health Ministers agreed that no progress could be made with it. The Commission was asked to bring forward a new version including a complete ban on press and poster advertising.

Tar yield

The EC Directive on the tar yield of manufactured cigarettes was adopted and legislation is being drafted. This Directive imposes a maximum tar yield of 15 mg in 1992, and 12 mg in 1997.

Smoking in public places

The EC Mixed Resolution on smoking in public places, accepted in 1989, recommends that Member States should ban smoking in public places, making provision for smokers where appropriate. This resolution will enable the UK to continue its current policy of encouraging the provision of smoke-free areas through voluntary means. The Government's White Paper on the Environment contained a commitment to issue guidance on smoking policies for public places.

(iii) Coronary heart disease

The Health Ministers adopted conclusions on coronary heart disease at their meeting in December 1990. These noted that the disease was a major cause of death in the working population. The Ministers recognised that a number of the preventive measures introduced against cancer also had a beneficial effect on heart disease, but considered that further measures could be identified and implemented. The Commission was asked to investigate the best way in which information exchanges and co-operation on national measures, including research and diagnosis, could be facilitated, and, in doing so, to make use of the assistance of experts and Member State representatives. The Commission was also asked to take account of the work of other bodies on the subject, particularly WHO.

(iv) Elderly people

In November 1990, the Council agreed to undertake a 3-year action programme to promote better understanding of the issues concerning elderly people, and to assist Member States in the development of their policies for this group. The emphasis of the programme is on the exchange of ideas and information to enable Member States to benefit from good practice and innovative ideas. Key objectives are to assist the development of preventive strategies to minimise dependency in later life; to promote better mutual understanding between the generations; and to assist the integration of older people in society—highlighting in particular the contribution they can make as much as the services they need. The establishment of a monitoring centre to enable information and research to be disseminated throughout the Community is proposed. It is also proposed to explore the possibility of setting up a network of innovative work in this field.

In implementing the decision of the Council, the Commission will be assisted by an advisory committee of representatives of the Member States, and it has appointed a number of expert external observers on whom it can call for advice. The UK Government is committed to playing a full and active role in the programme, and will wish to involve representatives of a number of statutory and voluntary agencies responsible for the provision of care for elderly people.

1993 has been designated 'European Year of the Elderly and of Solidarity between Generations', the activities for which will be decided during 1991.

(v) 'Europe Against Cancer'

An agreement in principle on the desirability of a 'Europe Against Cancer' initiative was reached in 1985. The overall aim of the programme was a reduction of 15% in expected cancer mortality by the year 2000. The main themes of the programme were:

- Prevention, including screening and anti-smoking measures.

- Public information and health education.

- Training of health professionals.

- Co-ordination of research.

A report on the implementation of the first action plan (1987–89) was issued in May 1990, and a second action plan for the years 1990–94, with a budget provision of up to 55 million ECU (around £38.5 million), was adopted. Its general aims are similar to those of the first action plan, and the specific heads of action are:

- Disseminating and monitoring the implementation of previous recommendations on cancer training for doctors, nurses and dentists.

- Encouraging mobility of students and professional staff.

- Promoting specific training projects.

- Exchanging experience of teaching materials, both in the general cancer field and with specific reference to palliative care.

The Department of Health (DH) has made contributions of £165,000 towards UK projects in support of this programme.

(vi) AIDS

On 17 May 1990, the Council of Health Ministers concluded that prevention by information, counselling and health education remained the priority in the campaign against the spread of HIV infection and AIDS. Recent progress in early intervention and treatment for people with HIV infection had resulted in improvements in health and an increase in life expectancy, and particular attention needed to be given to the future care needs of those infected. The Council also concluded that discrimination against HIV-seropositive people was an issue which should be given attention, and that a consistent approach for costing the management of care for infected people would assist financial forecasting in Member States.

The Council met again in November 1990 and invited Member States to promote access to early intervention and treatment in drug addiction services for drug misusers with HIV infection. It also invited Member States to extend their commitment to avoid discrimination to include those who live with, or work in contact with, people with HIV infection and AIDS. The Council invited the Commission to step up exchanges of information and experience on social and medical assistance for HIV-positive pregnant women, on systems of care for people with HIV infection and AIDS, and on the assessment of measures implemented in Member States to make safer injecting equipment available, including syringes and needles that can be used only once.

(vii) Manpower

In December 1990, as a result of the integration of the German Democratic Republic within the EC following the reunification of Germany, the Council adopted a new Directive covering the medical, dental and nursing professions. The Directive provides for Member States to recognise qualifications awarded in the former Republic on conditions similar to those applying to other EC nationals.

(viii) Movement of labour

EC Social Security Regulation 1408/71 continued to operate satisfactorily, providing health care cover for people moving between Member States. The major categories covered were temporary visitors, detached workers, and pensioners transferring their residence to another Member State. In 1990, 261 applications by UK patients for referral to other Member States specifically for treatment of pre-existing conditions were approved. About 360 citizens of other Member States were treated in the UK on the same basis. The incorporation of the former German Democratic Republic into the unified Germany extended activity under Regulation 1408/71 to the five new Lände of Germany.

(ix) Pharmaceuticals

During 1990, activity showed a marked increase as the deadline for completion of the single market, which includes pharmaceuticals, approached. Draft Directives on the rational use of medicines and on advertising, and the Commission's proposals to bring homoeopathic products within the scope of community law, and for future EC licensing arrangements, are described on pages 198–199.

(x) Medical devices

In June 1990 the Community adopted a Directive regulating the safety of powered implantable medical devices. It is the first of a series of three Directives to establish a European regulatory system for medical devices as part of the Community's plans for a single European market. The Directive covers a small range of high-technology implantable medical devices, such as cardiac pacemakers. The regulatory system in the Directive applies before the device is put on the market. Every device covered by it must comply with a series of essential requirements designed to ensure that each device:

– does not compromise the clinical condition of the patient;

– presents no risk to those implanting it; and

– achieves its intended performance.

In order to demonstrate that a product complies with these essential requirements, the manufacturer must have an approved quality control system covering design and production. Alternatively, he must submit a sample of the product for testing; this alternative route is supported by periodic sampling of production or, where appropriate, auditing of the production quality assurance system. In either case, the manufacturer undertakes to maintain post-marketing surveillance of his products. Devices fulfilling these requirements are entitled to bear a mark 'CE', signifying compliance with the Directive, and may be placed on the market of any Member State without further control. There are special provisions for custom-made devices, and for devices undergoing clinical investigation.

The Directive will be implemented by Regulations that must be in place by 1 July 1992 and take effect from 1 January 1993. There will be a transitional period of two years, ending on 31 December 1994, to allow manufacturers and regulatory authorities to adjust from existing national controls to the community system. Two other Directives are planned to make the Community's regulatory system comprehensive. The first, yet to be drafted, will cover in vitro diagnostic devices; the second, currently being drafted by the Commission, will cover all other medical devices.

(xi) Research and information technology

All EC research is carried out within the EC Research and Development Framework Programmes. The Second Framework Programme for the period 1987-91 is approaching completion, and a Third Framework Programme for the period 1990-94 has been agreed. The UK contributes 19% of the Framework Programme budgets. DH is closely involved in three specific research programmes within the Second Framework Programme, all of which will be carried forward to the Third Framework Programme.

The Medical and Health Research Programme 1987-91

The aim of the Medical and Health Research Programme 1987-91 (MHR4) is to achieve a 'critical mass' of researchers by bringing together their cumulative expertise to find solutions to medical or health problems of major EC importance. MHR4 is a programme of concerted actions, in which the EC funds the co-ordination costs only, the basic research being funded by the individual Member States. The Target Areas for MHR4 are cancer, AIDS, age-related health problems, environment and life-style related health problems, medical technology development, and health services research. The total cost of the 5-year programme is £44 million. The Department of Education and Science (DES) takes the UK lead, with DH providing support on a 60:40 basis to reflect the high biomedical content of the programme.

Biomedical and Health Research Programme 1990-94

Negotiations are being finalised for a new Biomedical and Health Research Programme 1990-94 (BIOMED I) within the Third Framework Programme. BIOMED I will be funded at a level of £90 million and the proposed Target Areas are:

- Development of co-ordinated research on prevention, care and health systems.

- Major health problems and diseases of great socio-economic impact (AIDS, cancer, cardiovascular disease, mental illness and neurological disease, ageing, age-related health problems and handicaps).

- Human Genome Analysis (HGA). This Target Area will subsume the Human Genome Analysis Programme 1990-91, which is treated as a separate research programme in the Second Framework Programme. HGA has a funding level of £10 million. DES and the Medical Research Council take the lead for the UK, with DH providing support on a 90:10 basis.

- Research on biomedical ethics.

Advanced Informatics in Medicine

Advanced Informatics in Medicine (AIM) is a programme of shared-cost research funding, in which successful proposals receive 50% of the research costs from the EC. It has the objective of securing the improvement of health care throughout Europe through the use of information technology and telecommunications. DH takes the UK lead, with the Department of Trade and Industry providing support on a 75:25 basis. The 2-year exploratory phase was funded to the level of £13 million under the Second Framework Programme. The main stage of AIM will be funded to the level of £68 million in the Third Framework Programme.

Radiation Protection

Radiation Protection (RPR) is a programme of shared-cost research funding with the objective of improving knowledge of human exposure to radiation. The funding for the 1990/91 RPR Programme was £14 million under the Second Framework Programme. The proposal for the 1992/93 RPR Programme, which will fall within the Third Framework Programme, is £19 million. DH takes 100% responsibility for this programme.

(xii) Nutrition—Recommended Daily Amounts

The Panel convened by the Committee on Medical Aspects of Food Policy (COMA) to review the Recommended Daily Amounts (RDA) for food energy and nutrients for groups of people in the UK completed its work during the year and its Report will be published early in 1991. One of the key uses of RDA is as a basis for nutritional labelling of foods. Following the issue of a Directive on nutrition labelling, this is now a major subject of EC interest, and, in 1990, the EC Scientific Committee for Food (SCF) set up its own review of RDA.

Two independent European scientists were initially appointed to the COMA Panel. At the request of the European Commission, the European representation on the COMA Panel was further strengthened by the appointment of two more observers from the SCF, and the Panel's draft Report was made available to the Commission. The Panel have gone beyond the old concept of RDA by defining a range of levels of nutrient intake called Dietary Reference Values (DRV). This has the advantage for labelling purposes of lessening the chance of misinterpretation of RDA as individual requirements for nutrients, when in fact they are almost always in excess of these. Estimated Average Requirements (EAR) have been defined; they can be more realistically interpreted as relevant to individual consumers, and should therefore not provoke unnecessary attempts by consumers to reach levels of nutrient intake which are virtually certain to be in excess of their requirements.

(c) Health Co-operation Agreements with Eastern Europe

The Health Co-operation Agreements which DH has with the USSR, Poland, Czechoslovakia, Hungary and, until reunification, the German Democratic Republic, provide a total of 145 weeks annually for UK specialists to visit these countries, and an equal number of weeks for specialists from these countries to visit the UK. The Agreements facilitate collaborative research, exchanges of specialists and delegations, the participation of experts in congresses and scientific conferences organised in the other country, and exchange of information on new equipment, pharmaceutical products and technological developments related to medicine and public health.

Co-operation is facilitated in the following fields of mutual interest:

USSR

Virology, oncology, ophthalmology, emergency medicine and traumatology, molecular biology approaches to brain mapping, rheumatology, diabetes mellitus, biomedical aspects of alcoholism and drug abuse, mother and child health care, organisation and provision of health services, primary care.

Poland

Cardiac surgery, neurosurgery, transplant immunology.

Czechoslovakia

Cardiac surgery, transplant surgery, cancer, tropical medicine, prevention and treatment of alcoholism, organisation and use of diagnostic laboratory services, screening for disease as an aspect of preventive medicine, organisation of outpatient services including primary care, postgraduate medical training.

Hungary

Organisation, planning and financing of health care services, primary health and community care, prevention of drug misuse, health education and information in the field of AIDS, organisation of health services.

German Democratic Republic

Anaesthesia, artificial organs and organ transplantation, oncology, laboratory diagnostics, communicable diseases, molecular biology, occupational health, diabetes, Alzheimer's disease and senile dementia, nursing methods, cardiovascular disease and preventive dentistry.

(d) WHO

(i) European Regional Committee

The 40th session of the WHO European Regional Committee was held in Copenhagen in September 1990. The UK delegation was led by the Chief Medical Officer for part of the meeting, and subsequently by Dr Jeremy Metters, Deputy Chief Medical Officer. The delegation included the Chief Medical Officer for Northern Ireland.

In his review of the health situation in Europe, the Regional Director referred to the political changes that were taking place. He stressed the need for increased support to be given to the new emerging democracies to help them restructure their health services, and redress the significant disparities in the health status of their populations. This led to the adoption by the Committee of a resolution to set up a programme for assistance to the countries concerned, with an appropriation of US $1 million from the Regular Budget for 1990/91 and US $2 million for 1992/93. In addition, an Advisory Sub-Committee was set up to advise on the programme, and to monitor its implementation. Other major developments discussed included the approval of the European Charter on Environment and Health, the development of the new concept of a generalist nurse, and the launching of a large scale initiative between the Regional Office and the International Diabetes Federation to implement a programme of diabetes control in Europe.

The revised procedure for the selection of the Regional Director for Europe by a Regional Search Group was approved. The budget proposals for 1992/93 were discussed and later accepted. However, many speakers expressed concern about the growing imbalance between expenditure on programmes and staff costs, and the trend towards an increase in extrabudgetary funds and their greater use for country programmes.

Although the Committee noted with satisfaction the progress made in increasing vaccination coverage in the Region, concern was expressed about the continuing outbreaks of poliomyelitis, diphtheria, measles, rubella and viral hepatitis in some Member States. Among the decisions taken was one requesting the Regional Director to develop a European Health for All information strategy. The technical discussions focused on healthy ageing. One of the major conclusions was that disease prevention programmes should include the elderly, as research had shown that elderly people could learn to avoid, and were able to resist, many diseases and the decline of functional capacity. It was possible to achieve a healthier life in old age within the limits defined by biological ageing.

(ii) Executive Board

In January 1990, the 85th session of the Executive Board was held under the chairmanship of Dr S Tapa, Minister of Health of Tonga. The Chief Medical Officer attended as the UK nominee on the Board.

In his address, the Director General listed a number of issues that would be given priority in the implementation of WHO's future programme of work. These included more attention to the consequences for human health of changes in the environment, the problem of widespread malnutrition and improper nutritional practices, and an emphasis on an integrated approach to disease control within primary health care. There was also to be a more realistic and pragmatic approach to the implementation of the primary health care approach. During the review of the Director General's report on drug dependence, the Chief Medical Officer announced the holding of a World Conference in London in April 1990 to reduce the demand for drugs and to combat the threat of cocaine. This was welcomed by the WHO Secretariat and members of the Board.

In the course of the various discussions, concern was expressed that insufficient attention was being given to unsustainable population growth, to the adverse effects on health of the deteriorating economy in developing countries, particularly the poorest, and to the continuing lack of primary health care structures in many countries. The complacency demonstrated by many governments and health professionals in implementing the International Code of Breast Milk Substitutes was criticised. However, the UK was singled out by the representative of the International Organisation of Consumers Unions for being one of the few countries to have taken effective measures to implement the Code.

The spread of the AIDS pandemic, and the devastating effect this was having in Africa, was repeatedly raised. Complacency about the disease was seen as one of the major threats to global health. The Chief Medical Officer called on WHO to take a stronger role in co-ordinating the efforts to find a vaccine. The deteriorating world-wide malaria situation received much attention and serious concern was expressed at the apparent lack of interest by the international community. The Chief Medical Officer proposed that WHO convene a global Conference of Ministers to help raise world consciousness about the situation.

His proposal received almost universal support from members of the Board, and the Director General promised to take the matter forward. Despite the fact that at least 1,000 million people were at risk of developing iodine deficiency disorders, the Board was impressed by the progress being made as a result of WHO's efforts. It set a target for the elimination of iodine deficiency disorders in all countries by the year 2000.

Professor H M Gilles was nominated for the award of the Darling Foundation Prize for his contribution in the field of malaria. Dr Jo Asvall and Dr Gottlieb Monekosso were re-elected Directors of the Regional Offices for Europe and Africa respectively, each for a further 5-year term.

(iii) World Health Assembly

The 43rd World Health Assembly was held in Geneva in May 1990. The UK delegation was led by the Secretary of State for part of the Assembly, and subsequently by the Chief Medical Officer, and Dr Jeremy Metters, Deputy Chief Medical Officer. The delegation included the Chief Nursing Officer and the Chief Medical Officer for Scotland.

President Mugabe of Zimbabwe and Mr Andreotti, the Italian President of the Council of Ministers, addressed the plenary session on the relationship between the world economy and health development. The major issues addressed by the Assembly included the problem of tobacco consumption, infant and young child nutrition, AIDS, malaria, and the serious problems facing the health sector in many developing countries because of the economic recession and debt repayments.

There was continuing consensus on the need to strengthen WHO's effort to reduce tobacco consumption, which was now being concentrated on stressing the dangers to health posed by smoke inhaled by non-smokers. Member States were encouraged to eliminate advertising and sponsorship of tobacco products, and to introduce progressive fiscal measures aimed at discouraging the use of tobacco.

The Assembly reiterated its concern over the decreasing prevalence and duration of breast feeding in many countries, and urged the promotion of breast feeding as an essential component of food and nutrition policies and programmes aimed at women and children. It resolved that WHO should aim at eliminating iodine deficiency disorders as a major health problem in all countries by the year 2000, and commended the establishment of a WHO Commission on Health and Environment to examine, inter alia, the subject of hazardous wastes and their potential effects on human health. Member States were urged to establish programmes for environmentally sound management of hazardous wastes, and to extend health surveillance, including epidemiological studies, to identify the adverse effects on populations of exposure to hazardous substances. The essential drugs list had been adopted in more than 100 countries, and some 50 countries had formulated national drug policies taking account of the WHO essential drug concept. Malaria was again one of the leading causes of morbidity and mortality in many tropical countries. The Assembly appealed to the pharmaceutical industry to increase its efforts to develop new drugs and vaccines for tropical diseases. The calling of an international Ministerial Conference on malaria was welcomed.

Discussion on AIDS underlined the changing patterns of the spread of the disease. Spread in Europe and the United States had shifted to intravenous drug misusers and the heterosexual community, whereas in Africa and some parts of South America spread through unsafe blood transfusions was still a major risk, in addition to heterosexual spread. The increased burden would fall on the hospital services in Africa, most of which were ill-equipped to cope even with their basic needs. This was a source of serious concern, as was the fate of the increasing number of orphans whose parents had died of AIDS. The crucial role of women, women's associations and non-governmental organisations in the prevention of HIV transmission and in the care of people with AIDS-related diseases was strongly emphasised. The appointment of Dr Michael Merson as the new Director of the WHO Programme on AIDS received the unanimous approval of all members of the Assembly. Generous tributes were paid to the previous Director, Dr J Mann, for his outstanding contribution to the programme.

The serious economic plight of many developing countries, especially the least developed, and its effects on the health sector, received much attention. Most delegates agreed that increased investment in health care would have to be preceded by substantial policy and management reforms. The action taken by WHO to intensify international technical co-operation to accelerate development of primary health care in the least developed countries was generally commended. A UK sponsored resolution on illicit drugs, stressing the importance of focusing on demand reduction, was adopted by consensus, and the Assembly approved the 10th International Classification of Diseases, which will come into force on 1 January 1991.

(e) Council of Europe

During the year the Committee of Ministers, on the recommendation of the European Health Committee, adopted recommendations on the impact of new technologies on health services, particularly primary health care, on training strategies for health information systems, on plasma products and European self-sufficiency, and on the protection of the mental health of certain vulnerable groups in society. It also adopted recommendations made by an ad hoc Committee on bioethics concerning medical research on human beings, and pre-natal genetic screening, genetic counselling and diagnosis. The 4th Council of Europe European Health Ministers' meeting was held in Cyprus in November 1990. It considered 'Health manpower: changes and challenges'. The UK was represented by Baroness Hooper, Parliamentary Under Secretary of State for Health (Lords).

Table A.1: *Population age and sex structure 1990, and changes by age, England, 1981-90*

Age (in years)	Resident population at mid-1990 (thousands)			Percentage changes (persons)			
	Persons	Males	Females	1981-90	1987-88	1988-89	1989-90
Under 1	648	332	316	8.3	3.2	-0.8	0.9
1-4	2542	1301	1240	13.7	1.5	2.5	1.1
5-15	6404	3287	3117	-14.0	-1.2	-0.6	0.6
16-29	10377	5283	5094	5.3	0.0	-0.5	-1.1
30-44	10031	5029	5002	9.3	0.8	0.7	1.0
45-64/59*	9040	5099	3941	-0.7	0.4	0.8	0.8
65/60-74**	5431	1883	3548	-3.7	-0.5	-0.5	-0.4
75-84	2625	966	1659	16.7	1.3	1.4	0.6
85+	740	188	551	44.6	4.7	5.0	3.9
All ages	47837	23368	24469	2.2	0.3	0.3	0.3

Note: figures may not add precisely to totals due to rounding.

* 45-64 years for males and 45-59 years for females.
** 65-74 years for males and 60-74 years for females.

Source: OPCS

Table A.2: *Five main causes of death at different ages (and percentages¹ of all causes of deaths), England, 1990*

RANK	All ages −1 and over Males	All ages −1 and over Females	1-14 Males	1-14 Females	15-34 Males	15-34 Females	35-54 Males	35-54 Females	55-74 Males	55-74 Females	75 and over Males	75 and over Females
1	Ischaemic heart disease	Ischaemic heart disease	Other causes of injury and poisoning†	Congenital anomalies	Road vehicle accidents	Other causes of injury and poisoning†	Ischaemic heart disease	MN* of bone, connective tissue, skin and breast	Ischaemic heart disease	Ischaemic heart disease	Ischaemic heart disease	Ischaemic heart disease
	30%	23%	18%	17%	26%	14%	29%	22%	35%	24%	27%	24%
2	Cerebro-vascular disease	Cerebro-vascular disease	Road vehicle accidents	Road vehicle accidents	Other causes of injury and poisoning†	Road vehicle accidents	MN* of digestive organs and peritoneum	MN* of genito-urinary organs	MN* of respiratory and intra-thoracic organs	MN* of digestive organs and peritoneum	Cerebro-vascular disease	Cerebro-vascular disease
	9%	15%	17%	14%	20%	13%	8%	11%	13%	9%	12%	17%
3	MN* of respiratory and intra-thoracic organs	MN* of digestive organs and peritoneum	Congenital anomalies	Other causes of injury and poisoning†	Suicide and self-inflicted injury	MN* of bone, connective tissue, skin and breast	MN* of respiratory and intra-thoracic organs	Ischaemic heart disease	MN* of digestive organs and peritoneum	Cerebro-vascular disease	Chronic obstructive pulmonary disease and allied conditions	Pneumonia
	9%	7%	12%	13%	16%	8%	8%	9%	10%	9%	8%	8%
4	MN* of digestive organs and peritoneum	Pneumonia	Diseases of the nervous system and sense organs	Diseases of the nervous system and sense organs	Diseases of the nervous system and sense organs	Suicide and self-inflicted injury	Other causes of injury and poisoning†	MN* of digestive organs and peritoneum	Cerebro-vascular disease	MN* of bone, connective tissue, skin and breast	MN* of respiratory and intra-thoracic organs	MN* of digestive organs and peritoneum
	8%	6%	10%	12%	5%	8%	8%	8%	7%	8%	7%	6%
5	MN* of genito-urinary organs	MN* of bone, connective tissue, skin and breast	MN* of lymphatic and haema-topoietic tissue	MN* of lymphatic and haema-topoietic tissue	MN* of lymphatic and haema-topoietic tissue	MN* of genito-urinary organs	Suicide and self-inflicted injury	Cerebro-vascular disease	Chronic obstructive pulmonary disease and allied conditions	MN* of respiratory and intra-thoracic organs	MN* of digestive organs and peritoneum	Mental disorders
	5%	5%	7%	5%	3%	5%	6%	6%	6%	8%	7%	6%
Remainder	39%	44%	36%	40%	30%	51%	41%	44%	30%	40%	39%	40%
All causes of death	256218	267460	1153	800	6402	2575	18006	11421	105996	71124	124661	181540

¹ May not add up to 100 due to rounding.
* MN = malignant neoplasm.
† 'Other causes of injury and poisoning' comprises categories of external injury and poisoning (E800-E999) excluding road vehicle accidents (E810-E829) and suicide (E950-E959).
Source: OPCS

223

Table A.3: Relative mortality from various conditions when presented as numbers of deaths and future years of 'working life' lost, England and Wales, 1989

Cause (ICD9 Code)	Males				Females			
	Number of deaths (thousands)		Years of 'working life' lost (thousands)		Number of deaths (thousands)		Years of 'working life' lost (thousands)	
	All ages	(%)	Age 15-64	(%)	All ages	(%)	Age 15-64	(%)
All causes, all ages	281		982		296		591	
All causes, 28 days and over	279	(100)	886	(100)	294	(100)	523	(100)
All malignant neoplasms* (140-208)	74	(27)	183	(21)	69	(24)	201	(38)
Lung cancer (162)	24	(9)	40	(4)	11	(4)	19	(4)
Breast cancer† (174)					14	(5)	62	(12)
Genito-urinary cancer (179-189)	13	(5)	15	(2)	10	(4)	39	(7)
Leukaemia (204-208)	2	(1)	15	(2)	2	(1)	10	(2)
Circulatory disease* (390-459)	127	(46)	220	(25)	137	(48)	77	(15)
Ischaemic heart disease (410-414)	83	(30)	158	(18)	68	(24)	34	(7)
Cerebrovascular disease (430-438)	25	(9)	28	(3)	42	(15)	23	(4)
Respiratory disease* (460-519)	33	(12)	42	(5)	33	(12)	28	(5)
Pneumonia (480-486)	10	(4)	13	(1)	18	(6)	8	(1)
Bronchitis, emphysema and asthma (490-493)	7	(2)	11	(1)	4	(1)	9	(2)
Sudden infant deaths (798.0)	1	(0)	36	(4)	0	(0)	23	(4)
All accidental deaths* (E800-E949)	7	(2)	153	(17)	5	(2)	43	(8)
Motor vehicle traffic accidents (E810-E819)	3	(1)	95	(11)	1	(0)	27	(5)
Suicide (E950-E959)	3	(1)	59	(7)	1	(0)	14	(3)

* These conditions are ranked as well as selected causes within these broader headings.

† Not calculated for male breast cancer.

Deaths under 28 days are excluded, except from 'All causes, all ages'.

Source: OPCS

224

Table A.4: *Trends in 'avoidable' deaths, England and Wales, 1979-89. Age standardised mortality ratios (1979 = 100)*

Condition	SMR[1]											Actual number of deaths[4]	
	1979	1980	1981	1982	1983	1984	1985	1986	1987	1988	1989	1979	1989
Hypertension/cerebrovascular (ages 35–64)	100	91	86	84	80	77	76	72	68	63	60	9482	5657
Perinatal mortality[2]	100	91	81	77	71	69	67	65	61	60	57	9400	5742
Cervical cancer (ages 15-64)	100	98	95	90	90	91	91	97	89	84	80	1142	910
Hodgkin's disease (ages 5-64)	100	99	99	86	86	79	75	74	82	74	64	365	246
Respiratory diseases (ages 1-14)	100	101	95	87	62	51	50	40	47	40	41	329	133
Surgical diseases[3] (ages 5-64)	100	87	81	77	71	78	66	72	53	69	52	262	134
Asthma (ages 5-44)	100	88	115	105	105	102	113	111	111	106	92	250	252
Tuberculosis (ages 5-64)	100	116	91	91	62	64	65	58	63	55	55	222	122
Chronic rheumatic heart disease (ages 5-64)	100	80	70	52	42	41	35	34	32	18	26	133	41
Total 'avoidable' deaths	100	92	85	81	76	74	72	70	66	62	59	21585	13237
All causes: ages 0-14	100	96	87	82	77	73	74	73	72	71	66	11132	7934
All causes: ages 15-64	100	96	93	92	90	88	88	86	84	82	80	127194	101092
All causes: all ages	100	96	95	94	93	89	92	89	86	85	85	591039	574938

[1] The standardised mortality ratio (SMR) for a condition is calculated by dividing the observed number of deaths by the expected number of deaths based on 1979 death rates.

[2] Stillbirths (3,232 in 1989) are included in perinatal mortality and total 'avoidable' deaths, but not in deaths from all causes.

[3] Appendicitis, abdominal hernia, cholelithiasis and cholecystitis.

[4] Excluding deaths of visitors to England and Wales.

Source: Calculated by Department of Health (SM12A) from data supplied by OPCS

Table A.5: *Live births, stillbirths, infant mortality and abortions, England, 1960-90*

| Year | Live births | Stillbirths | | Early neonatal mortality (deaths under 1 week) | | Perinatal mortality (stillbirths plus deaths under 1 week) | Post-neonatal mortality (deaths 4 weeks to under 1 year) | Infant mortality (deaths under 1 year) | Abortions[1] |
	Number	Number	Rate[2]	Number	Rate[3]	Rate[2]	Rate[3]	Rate[3]	Rate[4]
1960	740859	14753	19.5	9772	13.2	32.5	6.3	21.6	—
1970	741999	9708	12.9	7864	10.6	23.4	5.9	18.2	87.6
1975	563900	5918	10.4	5154	9.1	19.4	5.0	15.7	149.9
1976	550393	5339	9.6	4468	8.1	17.6	4.6	14.2	148.7
1977	536953	5087	9.4	4070	7.6	16.9	4.5	13.7	152.7
1978	562589	4791	8.4	3975	7.1	15.4	4.4	13.1	157.7
1979	601316	4811	7.9	4028	6.7	14.6	4.5	12.8	158.8
1980	619371	4523	7.3	3793	6.1	13.4	4.4	12.0	164.5
1981	598163	3939	6.5	3105	5.2	11.7	4.3	10.9	168.8
1982	589711	3731	6.3	2939	5.0	11.2	4.6	10.8	171.1
1983	593255	3412	5.7	2746	4.6	10.3	4.2	10.0	169.2
1984	600573	3425	5.7	2640	4.4	10.0	3.9	9.4	177.3
1985	619301	3426	5.5	2674	4.3	9.8	3.9	9.2	177.6
1986	623609	3337	5.3	2640	4.2	9.5	4.2	9.5	183.5
1987	643330	3224	5.0	2518	3.9	8.9	4.0	9.1	187.7
1988	654360	3188	4.8	2543	3.9	8.7	4.1	9.1	196.6
1989	649357	3056	4.7	2368	3.6	8.3	3.7	8.4	200.0
1990	666920	3068	4.6	2382	3.6	8.1	3.3	7.9	199.0

[1] Relates to England residents.
[2] Per 1,000 live and stillbirths.
[3] Per 1,000 live births.
[4] Per 1,000 conceptions (live births, stillbirths and abortions).

Source: OPCS

Table A.6: *Congenital malformations, England, 1980, 1985 and 1990*†

ICD Code(s)	Malformation		Stillbirths*			Live births**		
			1980	1985	1990	1980	1985	1990
	Malformed babies							
	Number		619	322	199	12704	12215	7520
	Rate		9.9	5.2	3.0	205.4	197.2	112.8
320-359, 740, 741, 742.0-742.5, 742.8, 742.9, 767.6	Central nervous system							
	Number		626	148	61	1087	679	299
	Rate		10.0	2.4	0.9	17.6	11.0	4.5
360-389, 743.0-743.6, 743.8-744.3	Ear and eye							
	Number		22	21	12	446	686	392
	Rate		0.4	0.3	0.2	7.2	11.1	5.9
749.0-749.2	Cleft lip/cleft palate							
	Number		49	19	17	815	758	691
	Rate		0.8	0.3	0.3	13.2	12.2	10.4
390-459, 745-747, 425.3, 745.4, 746.9, 747.0, 747.5, 747.9, 785.2	Cardiovascular							
	Number		16	12	21	817	794	558
	Rate		0.3	0.2	0.3	13.2	12.8	8.4
752.6	Hypospadias/epispadias							
	Number		1	3	1	930	1001	818
	Rate		0.0	0.0	0.0	15.0	16.2	12.3
755.0, 755.1	Polydactyly/syndactyly							
	Number		21	18	8	986	1097	912
	Rate		0.3	0.3	0.1	15.9	17.7	13.7
754.5-754.7	Talipes							
	Number		43	19	10	2318	1873	993
	Rate		0.7	0.3	0.1	37.5	30.2	14.9
758.0-758.9	Chromosomal							
	Number		16	16	21	523	520	472
	Rate		0.3	0.3	0.3	8.5	8.4	7.1

† From January 1990 certain minor malformations are no longer notified, and have been excluded from the figures shown. For example, club foot of positional origin is now excluded from the category 'Talipes', ICD Codes 754.5-754.7. This change in notification practice largely accounts for the decrease in the number of malformations reported in some categories in 1990.

* Rates per 10,000 total births.

** Rates per 10,000 live births.

Source: OPCS

227

Table A.7: *Cancer* registrations by sex, age and site: males, England and Wales, 1986*

Numbers and percentages

Age-group (years)

	All ages	%	0-14	%	15-24	%	25-44	%	45-64	%	65-74	%	75-84	%	85 and over	%
Eye, brain and other nervous system	1757	2	122	24	60	8	286	7	718	2	422	1	135	0	14	0
Mouth and pharynx	1791	2	6	1	13	2	103	2	759	3	515	1	327	1	68	1
Oesophagus	2591	3	0	0	1	0	58	1	803	3	915	3	681	2	133	2
Lung	24365	24	1	0	6	1	301	7	7017	24	9471	27	6542	23	1027	19
Stomach	6624	6	0	0	2	0	115	3	1719	6	2365	7	2038	7	385	7
Pancreas	2756	3	1	0	1	0	62	1	792	3	992	3	750	3	158	3
Large intestine and rectum	11710	11	1	0	14	2	327	8	3287	11	3989	11	3417	12	675	13
Prostate	10180	10	0	0	1	0	15	0	1301	4	3818	11	4146	15	899	17
Bladder	6781	7	2	0	13	2	164	4	1914	7	2425	7	1916	7	347	6
Skin	15141	15	11	2	53	7	828	20	4741	16	4954	14	3765	13	789	15
Leukaemias and lymphomas	6445	6	253	49	313	40	692	17	1834	6	1679	5	1383	5	291	5
All other cancer	13354	13	118	23	302	39	1238	30	4087	14	4094	11	2941	10	574	11
Total cancer	103495	100	515	100	779	100	4189	100	28972	100	35639	100	28041	100	5360	100

* Cancer = malignant neoplasm.

Source: OPCS

Table A.8: *Cancer* registrations by sex, age and site: females, England and Wales, 1986*

Numbers and percentages

Age-group (years)

	All ages		0-14		15-24		25-44		45-64		65-74		75-84		85 and over	
		%		%		%		%		%		%		%		%
Eye, brain and other nervous system	1312	1	97	24	60	9	192	2	482	2	310	1	148	1	23	0
Mouth and pharynx	996	1	2	0	9	1	74	1	287	1	292	1	247	1	85	1
Oesophagus	1812	2	0	0	0	0	21	0	354	1	523	2	647	2	267	3
Breast	22757	22	3	1	22	3	2963	37	9053	30	5296	19	3985	15	1435	15
Lung	9991	10	1	0	2	0	185	2	2976	10	3739	14	2487	10	601	6
Stomach	4029	4	0	0	2	0	64	1	608	2	1058	4	1606	6	691	7
Pancreas	2831	3	1	0	1	0	37	0	508	2	863	3	1022	4	399	4
Large intestine and rectum	12393	12	1	0	7	1	298	4	2815	9	3379	12	4093	16	1800	19
Ovary	4507	4	8	2	48	8	415	5	1795	6	1210	4	815	3	216	2
Cervix	4034	4	1	0	42	7	1452	18	1369	5	696	3	359	1	115	1
Other uterus	3812	4	0	0	2	0	140	2	1615	5	1074	4	750	3	231	2
Bladder	2810	3	5	1	5	1	49	1	659	2	888	3	879	3	329	3
Skin	14428	14	14	3	96	15	1115	14	3543	12	3901	14	4175	16	1584	16
Leukaemias and lymphomas	5434	5	157	39	206	32	488	6	1221	4	1363	5	1479	6	520	5
All other cancer	11163	11	117	29	134	21	584	7	2626	9	3023	11	3326	13	1353	14
Total cancer	102309	100	403	100	636	100	8077	100	29911	100	27615	100	26018	100	9649	100

* Cancer = malignant neoplasm.

Source: OPCS

229

Table A.9: *Numbers (in thousands) of children aged 16 years and under completing primary course of immunisation with the percentage of eligible children immunised by the end of the second year after birth in brackets. For BCG this percentage is the estimated school population aged 13 years who were immunised in the year. England, 1976-89/90*

Year	Diphtheria		Tetanus		Polio		Whooping cough		Measles		BCG	
1976	487.5	(75)	510.2	(75)	495.6	(75)	240.6	(38)	323.7	(47)	564.4	(74)
1977	490.9	(78)	513.1	(78)	515.6	(78)	191.9	(40)	304.9	(50)	590.1	(76)
1978	506.0	(78)	524.4	(79)	518.8	(78)	199.4	(31)	302.1	(48)	576.6	(74)
1979	528.6	(80)	543.7	(80)	533.6	(80)	250.3	(35)	331.7	(51)	563.9	(74)
1980	545.9	(81)	560.2	(81)	549.7	(81)	285.6	(41)	351.6	(53)	617.9	(82)
1981	552.2	(83)	564.4	(83)	554.5	(82)	320.5	(46)	368.5	(55)	575.1	(78)
1982	558.1	(84)	572.7	(84)	562.8	(84)	384.8	(53)	390.7	(58)	547.1	(75)
1983	528.5	(84)	538.3	(84)	531.5	(84)	406.8	(59)	392.9	(60)	539.8	(76)
1984	532.1	(84)	540.2	(84)	534.0	(84)	391.7	(65)	435.6	(63)	507.9	(71)
1985	544.4	(85)	551.6	(85)	548.9	(85)	414.2	(65)	473.8	(68)	518.7	(77)
1986	563.6	(85)	573.1	(85)	569.1	(85)	475.9	(67)	502.9	(71)	486.7	(76)
1987/88[1]	701.4	(87)	709.7	(87)	703.8	(87)	590.3	(73)	647.3	(76)	450.2	(76)
1988/89[2]	603.5	(87)	644.0	(87)	606.8	(87)	517.3	(75)	1005.2[3]	(80)	408.8	(71)
1989/90[2]	642.6	(89)	690.5	(89)	649.5	(89)	581.8	(78)	1396.0[3]	(84)	197.4	(36)[4]

[1] Figures for 1987/88 are not directly comparable with previous years due to the change to recording figures for the year April-March. They cover the 15 month period between 1 January 1987 and 31 March 1988, with the exception of the figures for BCG which cover the period 1 April 1987 to 31 March 1988.

[2] Figures for 1988/89 onwards are for the period 1 April to 31 March. The uptake rate for this period is the percentage of children immunised by their second birthday. The numbers presented include some adults over 16 years-of-age who completed a primary course of immunisation.

[3] The number immunised against measles in 1988/89 and 1989/90 includes children who received MMR vaccine and who had already received single antigen measles vaccine.

[4] The school BCG programme was suspended in 1989 because there were insufficient supplies of BCG vaccine.

Sources: 1976-87/88: Form SBL 607 (Department of Health)
1988/89 and 1989/90: Forms KC50 and KC51 (Department of Health)

230

Table A.10: *Cumulative totals of AIDS cases by exposure category, England, to 31 December 1990*

(Numbers subject to revision as further data are received or duplicates identified)

How persons probably acquired the virus	Number of cases			%†
	Male	Female	Total	
Sexual intercourse				
between men	3086	0	3086	81
between men and women				
'high risk' partner*	11	17	28	1
other partner abroad**	128	59	187	5
other partner UK	10	12	22	1
Injecting drug use (IDU)	77	24	101	3
IDU and sexual intercourse				
between men	60	0	60	2
Blood				
Blood factor (eg haemophiliacs)	202	3	205	5
Blood or tissue transfer (eg transfusion)	24	37	61	2
Mother to child	15	17	32	1
Other/undetermined	31	4	35	1
Total	3644	173	3817	100

* Includes men and women who had sex with injecting drug users, or with those infected by contaminated blood, and women who had sex with bisexual men.

** Includes persons without other identified risks who are from, or who have lived in, countries where the major route of HIV1 transmission is through sexual intercourse between men and women.

† Total does not add up to 100 because of rounding.

Source: CDSC

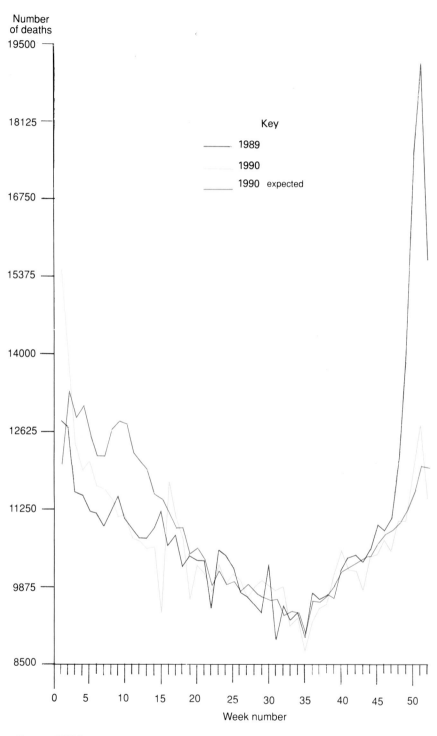

Source: OPCS

Printed in the United Kingdom for HMSO
Dd295201 9/91 C21 G3392 10170